Demos Surgical Pathology Guides

Liver Pathology

Demos Surgical Pathology Guides

SERIES EDITOR

Saul Suster, MD
Professor and Chairman
Department of Pathology
Medical College of Wisconsin
Milwaukee, Wisconsin

TITLES

- ***Head and Neck Pathology***
  Paul E. Wakely
- ***Breast Pathology***
  Giovanni Falconieri, Janez Lamovec, and Abiy B. Ambaye
- ***Inflammatory Skin Disorders***
  Jose A. Plaza and Victor G. Prieto
- ***Lymph Nodes***
  Horatiu Olteanu, Alexandra M. Harrington, and Steven H. Kroft
- ***Neoplastic Lesions of the Skin***
  Jose A. Plaza and Victor G. Prieto
- ***Pulmonary Pathology***
  Nagarjun Rao and Cesar A. Moran
- ***Prostate Pathology***
  Debra L. Zynger and Anil V. Parwani
- ***Liver Pathology***
  Shu-Yuan Xiao and Kiyoko Oshima

Demos Surgical Pathology Guides

Liver Pathology

SHU-YUAN XIAO, MD
Professor of Pathology
University of Chicago Medical Center
Chicago, Illinois

KIYOKO OSHIMA, MD
Associate Professor of Pathology
Medical College of Wisconsin
Milwaukee, Wisconsin

demosMEDICAL
New York

Visit our website at www.demosmedical.com

ISBN: 9781620700075
e-book ISBN: 9781617051715

Acquisitions Editor: Rich Winters
Compositor: diacriTech

Medicine is an ever-changing science. Research and clinical experience are continually expanding our knowledge, in particular our understanding of proper treatment and drug therapy. The authors, editors, and publisher have made every effort to ensure that all information in this book is in accordance with the state of knowledge at the time of production of the book. Nevertheless, the authors, editors, and publisher are not responsible for errors or omissions or for any consequences from application of the information in this book and make no warranty, expressed or implied, with respect to the contents of the publication. Every reader should examine carefully the package inserts accompanying each drug and should carefully check whether the dosage schedules mentioned therein or the contraindications stated by the manufacturer differ from the statements made in this book. Such examination is particularly important with drugs that are either rarely used or have been newly released on the market.

Library of Congress Cataloging-in-Publication Data

Xiao, Shu-Yuan.
Liver pathology / Shu-Yuan Xiao, MD, Professor of Pathology, University of Chicago Medical Center, Chicago, Illinois, Kiyoko Oshima, MD, Associate Professor of Pathology, Medical College of Wisconsin, Milwaukee, Wisconsin.
pages; cm. — (Demos surgical pathology guides)
Includes bibliographical references and index.
ISBN 978-1-62070-007-5
1. Liver—Diseases. I. Oshima, Kiyoko. II. Title.
RC846.9.X53 2014
616.3'62—dc23

2014014116

Printed in the United States of America by Bradford and Bigelow.
14 15 16 17 / 5 4 3 2 1

Contents

Series Foreword

The field of surgical pathology has gained increasing relevance and importance over the years as pathologists have become more and more integrated into the health care team. To the need for precise histopathologic diagnoses has now been added the burden of providing our clinical colleagues with information that will allow them to assess the prognosis of the disease and predict the response to therapy. Pathologists now serve as key consultants in the patient management team and are responsible for providing critical information that will guide their therapy. With the progress gained due to the insights obtained from the application of newer diagnostic techniques, surgical pathology has become progressively more complex. As a result, diagnoses need to be more detailed and specific and the number of data elements required in the generation of a surgical pathology report have increased exponentially, making management of the information required for diagnosis cumbersome and sometimes difficult.

The past 15 years have witnessed an explosion of information in the field of pathology with a massive proliferation of specialized textbooks appearing in print. For the most part, such texts provide in-depth and detailed coverage of the various areas in surgical pathology. The purpose of this series is to bridge the gap between the major subspecialty texts and the large, double-volume general surgical pathology textbooks, by providing compact, single-volume monographs that will succinctly address the most salient and important points required for the diagnosis of the most common conditions. The series is organized following an organ-system format, with single volumes dedicated to individual organs. The volumes are divided on the basis of disease groups, including benign reactive, inflammatory, infectious or systemic conditions, benign neoplastic conditions, and malignant neoplasms. Each chapter consists of a bulleted list of the most pertinent clinical data related to the condition, followed by the most important histopathologic criteria for diagnosis, pertinent use of immunohistochemical stains and other ancillary techniques, and relevant molecular tests when available. This is followed by a section on differential diagnosis. References appear at the back of the volume. Each entity is illustrated with key, high-quality histological images that highlight the most salient and distinctive features that need to be recognized for the correct diagnosis.

These books are intended for the busy practicing pathologist, and for pathology residents and fellows in training who require an easy and simple overview of major diagnostic criteria and key points during the course of routine daily practice. The authors have been carefully chosen for their experience in the field and clarity of exposition in the various topics. It is hoped that this series will fulfill its purpose of providing quick and easy access to critical information for the busy practitioner or trainee, and that it will assist pathologists in their routine practice of the specialty.

Saul Suster, MD
Professor and Chairman
Department of Pathology
Medical College of Wisconsin
Milwaukee, Wisconsin

Preface

While some medical liver diseases have diagnostically characteristic histologic features, there are many others for which proper diagnosis can only be achieved by close integration of clinical history, laboratory data, and microscopic analysis of a biopsy specimen. For example, in a biopsy that exhibits chronic hepatitis with interface activity, the differential diagnosis would include chronic viral hepatitis of various etiologies, autoimmune hepatitis, Wilson's disease, and even drug-induced liver injury. Although there are additional specific histologic features for some diseases, such as marked plasma cell infiltration and brisk interface activity in autoimmune hepatitis, ballooned periportal hepatocytes with copper accumulation in Wilson's disease, prominent portal lymphoid follicles in hepatitis C, etc., these features are not always present in the biopsy. Therefore, correlation with relevant clinical history and laboratory tests is crucial.

Another challenging issue in the proper interpretation of liver biopsy pathology is the presence of two disease processes in the same biopsy. For instance, nonalcoholic fatty liver disease often co-exists with chronic hepatitis C. The proper grading and staging of these two processes can be problematic since there are some features of necroinflammatory activity (grade) and fibrosis (stage) that are unique to each disease state, but others that overlap to a significant extent. The proper role of the surgical pathologist is to attempt to assign the most significant histologic features to the proper disease state and provide guidance to the treating clinician as to which process is primarily responsible for the ongoing liver injury. In some circumstances, this may be very difficult or even impossible. Histologic interpretation of liver allograft biopsies is particularly fraught with such issues, since there are a myriad of possible overlapping immunologic, surgical, therapeutic, and infectious insults to the graft.

As the above examples suggest, proper histologic examination of a liver biopsy specimen frequently requires a working knowledge of the fundamentals of hepatology and clinical pathology, so that clinical features and laboratory data can be incorporated into a final diagnosis. As such, this volume of simple bullet-pointed text and photomicrographs is not intended as a definitive resource. Rather, we intend this volume to serve as a practical reference guide for the practicing surgical pathologist during daily diagnostic work. Our aim is to provide residents, fellows, and medical students an up-to-date overview of liver diseases of current clinical relevance with concise information helpful in establishing first a differential diagnosis and then, where possible, a final diagnosis which includes the information most helpful for guiding proper clinical management.

Although there are many reasonable ways to organize the information provided in this text, there is clearly no perfect system and some degree of repetition and overlap is unavoidable, and may even be of benefit to the reader. We have attempted to provide the information in as user-friendly a fashion as we could devise, with the intent of placing information where a busy practicing surgical pathologist would most likely look for it when considering a given difficult biopsy specimen.

Acknowledgment

We'd like to thank Dr. Saul Suster, the series editor for trusting us with this task, and Mr. Rich Winters of Demos Medical Publishing for his professional guidance and assistance in the production of this volume. We also thank Drs. Lindsay Alpert and Lei Zhao for their critical reading of the chapters. Dr. Xiuli Liu graciously provided images for some of the chapters, for which we are grateful.

Personal note from Shu-Yuan Xiao: I would like to thank my mentor, Dr. John Hart, who taught me liver pathology. My family, Fang, Stephanie, and Emily have always been here to support me; without their encouragement I wouldn't have started this project.

Demos Surgical Pathology Guides

Liver Pathology

1

Acute Hepatitis and Fulminant Hepatic Failure

FULMINANT HEPATIC FAILURE

ACUTE HEPATOTROPIC VIRAL INFECTIONS

OTHER INFECTIOUS HEPATITIDES

FIBROSING CHOLESTATIC HEPATITIS

DRUG-INDUCED HEPATIC NECROSIS

PREGNANCY-RELATED ACUTE HEPATITIS

Fulminant Hepatic Failure

DEFINITION

Potentially reversible severe liver dysfunction developing in 8 weeks or less from the initial symptom with no prior history of liver disease

CLINICAL FEATURES

- Encephalopathy, coagulopathy.
- Emergency transplantation may be indicated.
- Etiologies include acetaminophen toxicity (46%), idiosyncratic reaction to other drugs (11%), hepatitis B (7%) (Figure 1-1A), hepatitis A (3%), autoimmune hepatitis (5%) (Figure 1-1B), ischemia (4%), Wilson's disease (2%), others (7%), or unknown etiology (14%).
- Serologic studies generally required to identify etiology.

PATHOLOGIC FINDINGS

- Massive hepatic necrosis: confluent necrosis throughout the liver; liver size and weight reduced by one-half to two-thirds.
- Sub-massive necrosis: course more protracted, liver forms regenerative nodules (Figures 1-1C, D).
- Recognition and diagnosis of autoimmune hepatitis (central venulitis, plasma cell infiltrate, interface hepatitis) crucial due to available treatment by immunosuppressive therapy.
- Zonal distribution of necrosis helpful in identifying etiology: zone 3 necrosis favoring acetaminophen toxicity; zone 2 necrosis traditionally reported in yellow fever; zone 1 necrosis suggestive of hepatitis A.

DIFFERENTIAL DIAGNOSIS

- Prior history of viral hepatitis
- Exacerbation of known autoimmune hepatitis

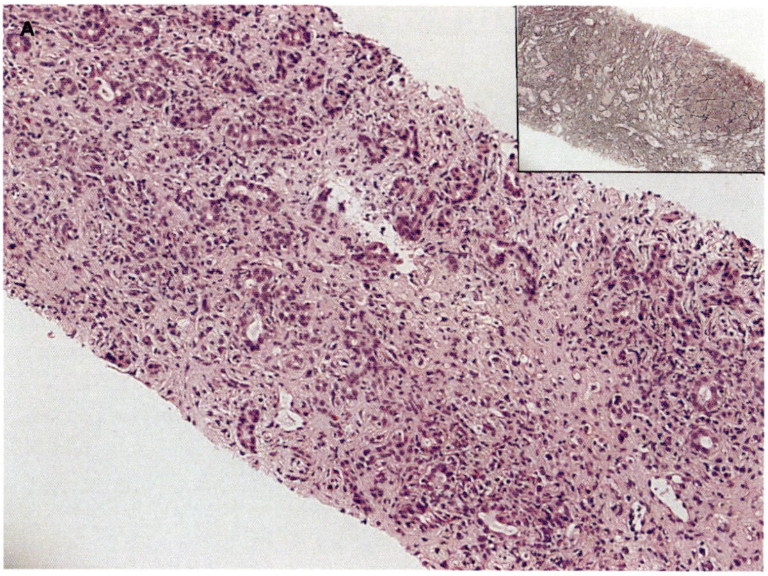

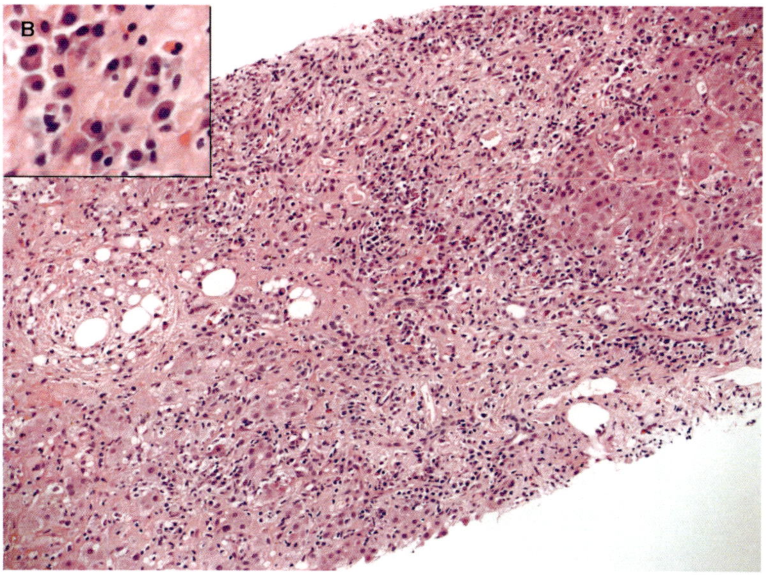

FIGURE 1-1

FIGURE 1-1 (A) Fulminant hepatic failure due to HBV: normal parenchyma replaced by collapsed fibrous stroma with proliferating bile ductules. The histologic appearance is not specific. Reticulin stain highlights collapse (insert). (B) Fulminant hepatic failure due to autoimmune hepatitis. There is extensive necrosis with marked plasma cell infiltrate (insert).

(*continued*)

Fulminant Hepatic Failure *(continued)*

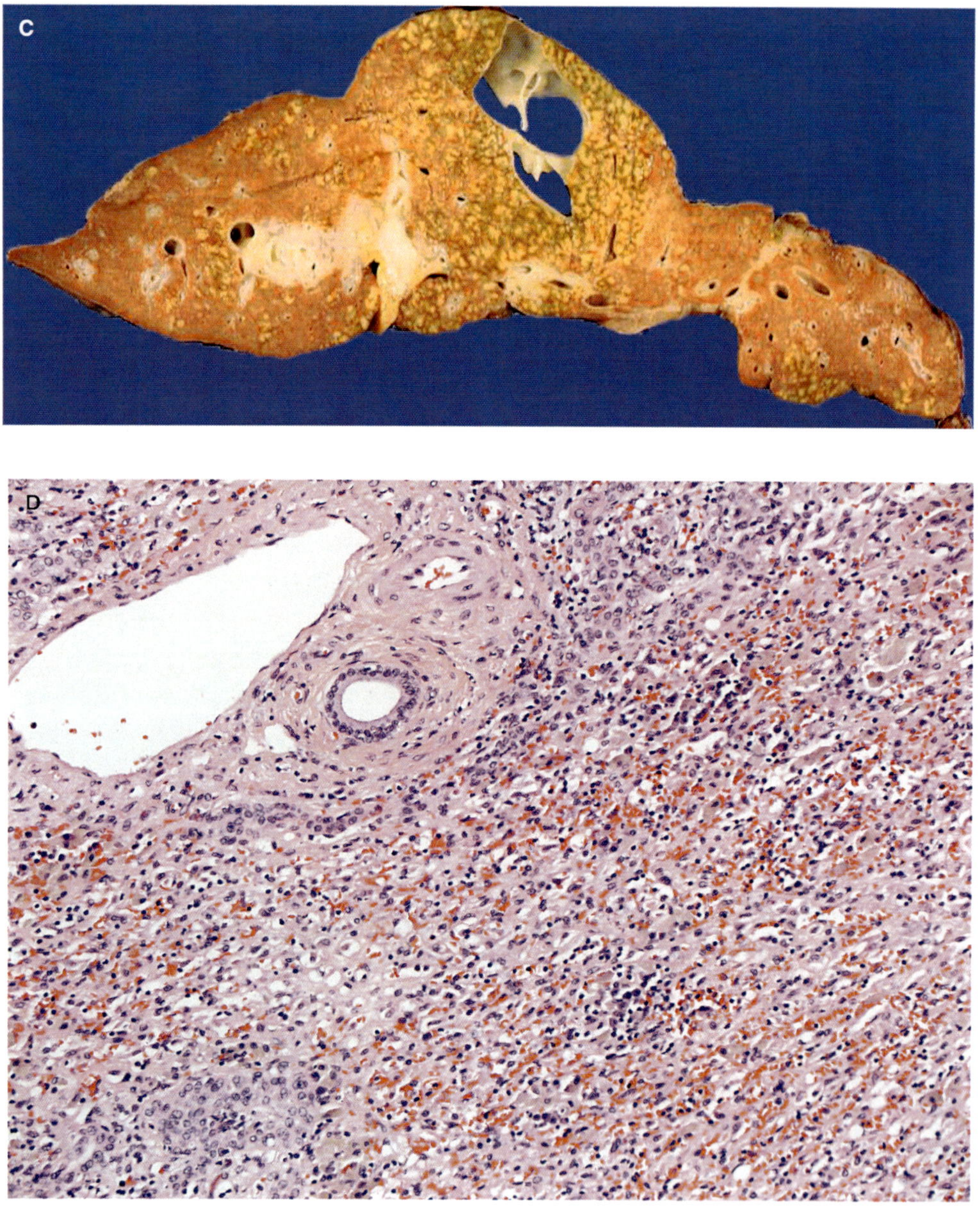

FIGURE 1-1

FIGURE 1-1 (C) Sub-massive necrosis of unknown etiology. Regenerative nodules are evident in the center of the specimen. The brown areas in the right and left represent parenchyma collapse. (D) Extensive, near-total hepatocyte necrosis, leaving behind sinusoidal stroma, and intact unremarkable portal tract (left upper corner).

Acute Hepatotropic Viral Infections

DEFINITION

Elevation of ALT and/or AST caused by one of the hepatotropic viruses (A to G) in a patient without a previous history of liver disease

CLINICAL FEATURES

- Severity varies from a mild asymptomatic infection to fatal fulminant hepatic failure.
- Serology confirms diagnosis; liver biopsy usually not necessary except to rule out secondary contributing factors or atypical clinical presentation.
- Hepatitis A or E rarely progresses to chronic hepatitis.
- Hepatitis C is usually asymptomatic in acute phase.
- Hepatitis Delta requires coinfection with HBV.
- Hepatitis E is endemic in Indian subcontinent; however, recently non-travel-associated hepatitis E has been reported in industrialized countries.

HISTOLOGIC FINDINGS

- Acute hepatitis is characterized by lobular disarray due to hepatocellular damage, swelling, and concurrent regeneration (Figures 1-2A, B). Frequent microscopic changes include ballooning degeneration, scattered acidophil bodies, hepatocytes dropout, lobular and sinusoidal inflammatory cell infiltrate, and Kupffer cell hyperplasia (Figure 1-2C).
- Zonal and bridging necrosis indicates a greater risk for developing fibrosis.
- Acute hepatitis in resolving phase can be subtle, and increased PASD positive histiocytes may be the only finding (Figure 1-2D).

DIFFERENTIAL DIAGNOSIS

- Drug-related liver injury
- Autoimmune hepatitis
- Acute alcoholic hepatitis

(continued)

Acute Hepatotropic Viral Infections *(continued)*

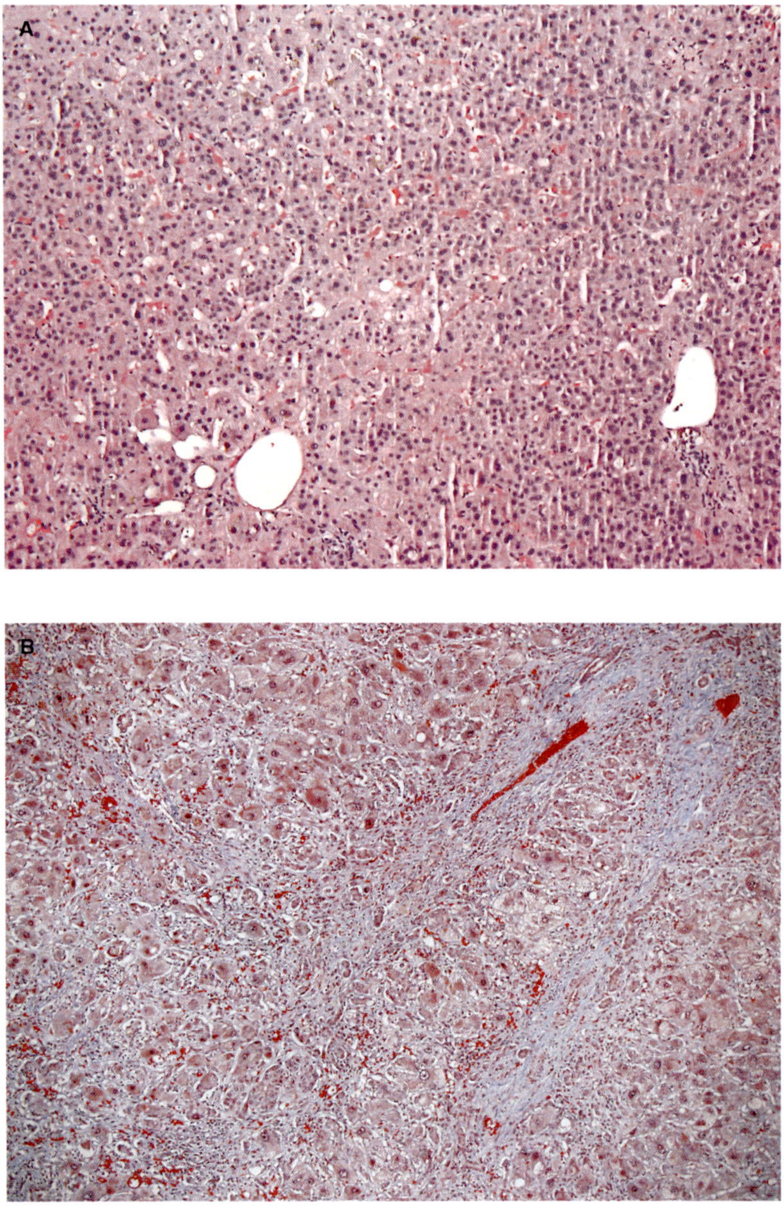

FIGURE 1-2

FIGURE 1-2 (A) Acute hepatitis with lobular disarray due to increased regenerative activity and swelling of hepatocytes. (B) Trichrome stain shows no significant fibrosis. Edematous areas with light staining are indicative of collapsed framework.

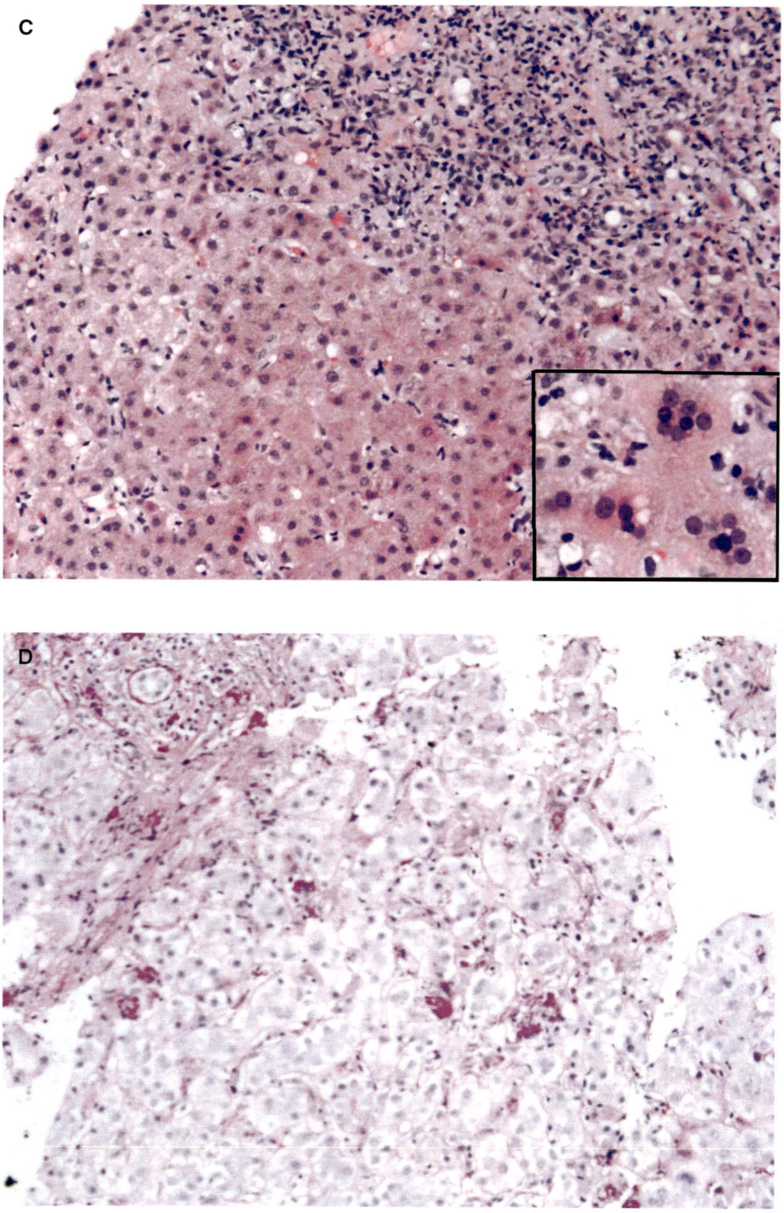

FIGURE 1-2

FIGURE 1-2 (C) Acute hepatitis A. Lobular disarray with loss of normal trabecular pattern. Portal lymphoplasmacytic infiltrate with interface activity. Multinucleated giant cells are present in the lobules as well (insert). (D) Resolving acute hepatitis A. PASD highlights increased PAS positive macrophages (phagocytosed cellular debris).

Other Infectious Hepatitides

DEFINITION

Acute hepatitis due to nonhepatotropic viruses such as Epstein-Barr virus (EBV), cytomegalovirus (CMV), herpes simplex virus (HSV), varicella-zoster virus (VZV), and yellow fever virus (YFV)

CLINICAL FEATURES

- EBV is a member of herpesvirus family and causes hepatitis and lymphoproliferative disorders. Infectious mononucleosis typically occurs in adolescents or young adults and presents with fevers, fatigue, malaise, sore throat, jaundice, and lymphadenopathy.
- Most CMV infections are clinically silent. Clinically significant infections are seen in setting of immunosuppression (organ transplantation, acquired immunodeficiency, and congenital infection).
- HSV hepatitis is seen in neonates, pregnant women, and immunocompromised patients. Immune competent individuals may rarely develop fulminant infection.
- Yellow fever still occurs in people travelling to tropical regions without proper vaccination or rarely as a small outbreak due to vaccine adverse effect.

PATHOLOGIC FEATURES

- Herpes hepatitis: nonzonal coagulative necrosis, eosinophilic intranuclear inclusions surrounded by halo (Cowdry Type A), multinucleated cells with molding (Figure 1-3A).
- Cytomegaloviral hepatitis: cytoplasmic and nuclear enlargement with intranuclear and intracytoplasmic inclusions, neutrophilic microabscesses formation; microgranuloma may be seen (Figure 1-3B).
- EBV hepatitis: diffuse sinusoidal infiltration by lymphocytes in string of beads pattern (Figure 1-3C).
- Yellow fever viral hepatitis: focal or confluent hepatic coagulative necrosis.

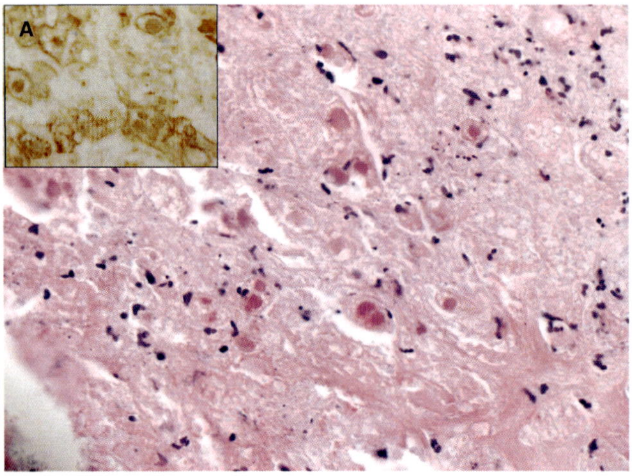

FIGURE 1-3

FIGURE 1-3 (A) HSV hepatitis. Inclusions characterized by smudged nuclei are seen in the setting of extensive hepatic necrosis; some inclusions are multinucleated. Immunohistochemical staining (insert) for both HSV1 and HSV2 should be performed.

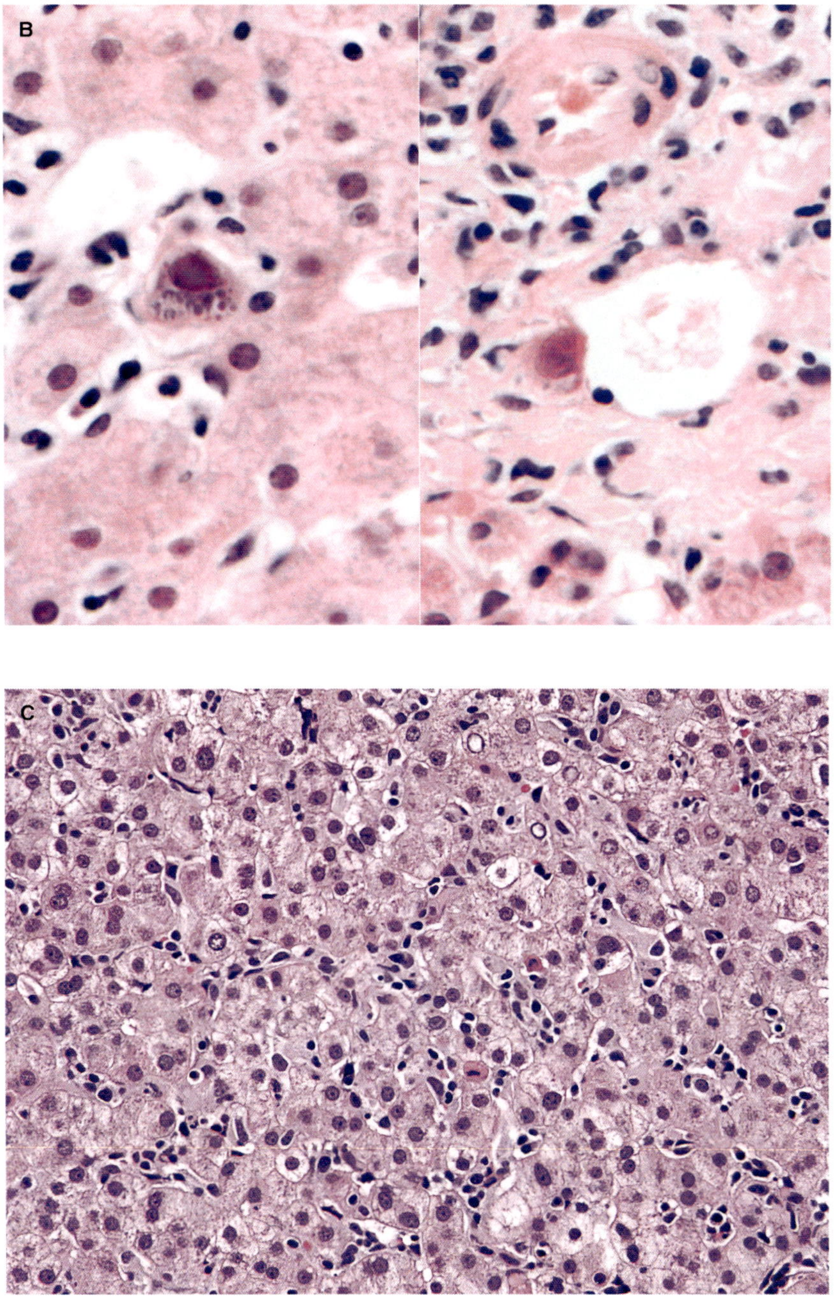

FIGURE 1-3

FIGURE 1-3 (B) CMV hepatitis. A hepatocyte with an enlarged nucleus; intranuclear and intracytoplasmic inclusions are present in the hepatocyte (left), and in an endothelial cell of the portal vein (right). Inclusions can be seen in biliary epithelium or Kupffer cells as well. (C) EBV hepatitis. Diffuse sinusoidal lymphocytic infiltration in string of beads pattern, with occasional acidophil bodies.

Fibrosing Cholestatic Hepatitis

DEFINITION

A rare form of aggressive hepatitis occurring in immunocompromised or immune suppressed patients that is associated with poor outcome. Though originally reported in liver transplant recipients with recurrent hepatitis B, this entity has now been recognized to occur in chronic hepatitis B or C patients who are under immunosuppression or have HIV co-infection.

CLINICAL FEATURES

- Most patients diagnosed within the first year post-liver transplant.
- High serum transaminase elevation, increased bilirubin, and jaundice.
- High viral load.

PATHOLOGIC FEATURES

- Extensive portal fibrosis with delicate septa extending into sinusoids (perisinusoidal fibrosis) (Figure 1-4A).
- Marked canalicular and hepatocellular cholestasis with ballooning (Figure 1-4B).
- Minimal to mild inflammatory cellular infiltration.

DIFFERENTIAL DIAGNOSIS

- Biliary obstruction

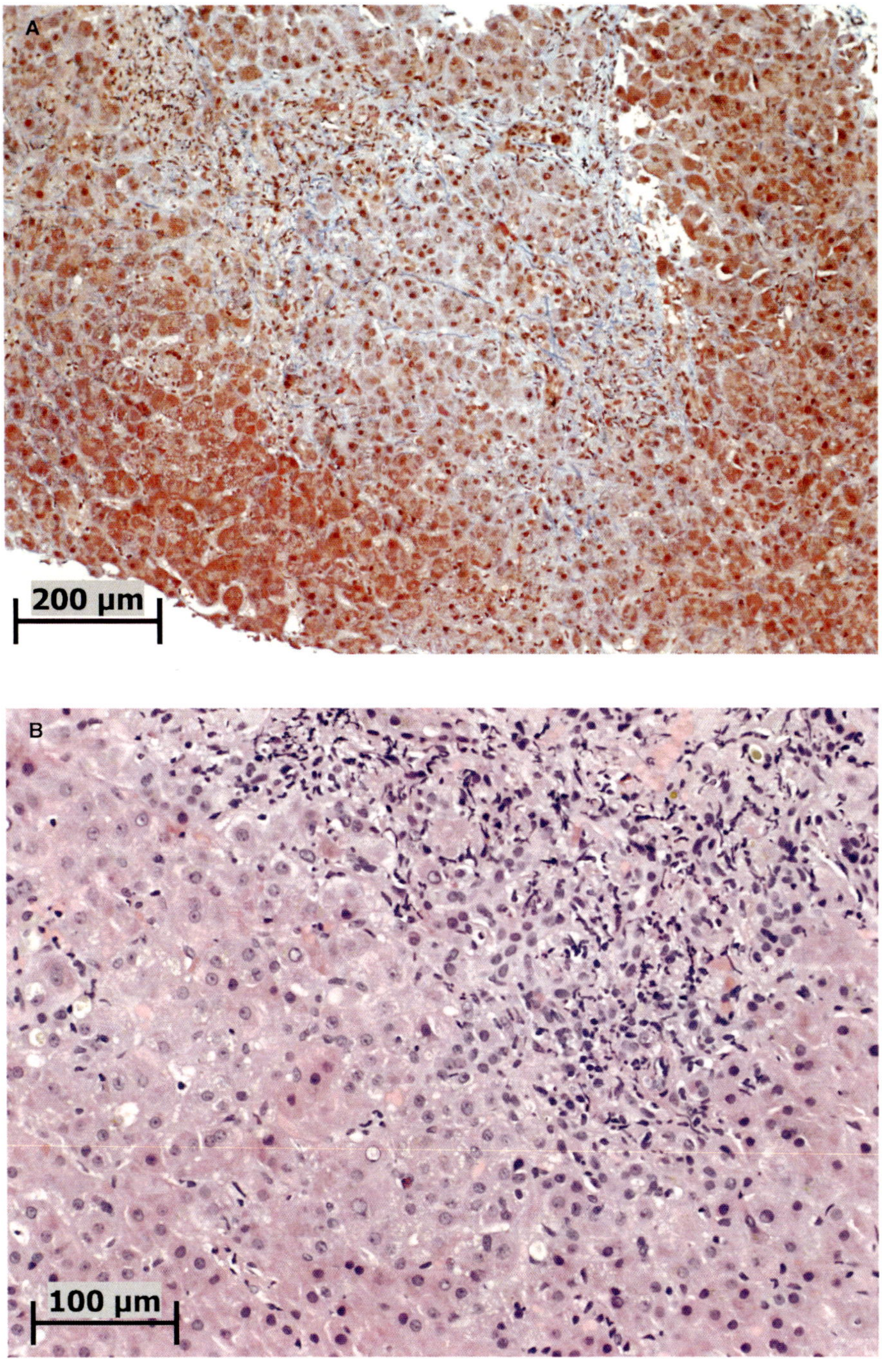

FIGURE 1-4

FIGURE 1-4 (A) Extensive portal fibrosis with delicate septa extending into sinusoids. (B) Fibrosing cholestatic recurrent hepatitis C. Bile ductular proliferation and hepatocyte ballooning, with minimal inflammatory infiltrates.

Drug-Induced Hepatic Necrosis

DEFINITION

Sudden abnormality of liver biochemical tests (alanine aminotransferase, alkaline phosphatase and/or bilirubin) with underlying liver necrosis related to intake of drug or toxin

CLINICAL FEATURES

- Typically present with new onset of abnormal LFTs, with no causes identifiable by clinical history and serology.
- Patterns of liver enzyme abnormality classified as hepatic type, cholestatic type, or mixed type.
- Hepatotoxic agents sub-classified into 2 groups: (1) intrinsic toxins that are dose dependent and reproducible, such as acetaminophen (Figure 1-5A); (2) idiosyncratic toxins that are not dose dependent and are unpredictable, such as isoniazid (Figures 1-5B, C).
- Obtaining drug history and a literature search for each drug the patient is taking is necessary to confirm the diagnosis in suspected cases.
- Measurement of serum level of drug helpful but may be noncontributory due to metabolism.
- Antinuclear or anti-smooth muscle antibodies may be present.
- Normalization of liver enzymes takes weeks or months after the drug is stopped.

PATHOLOGIC FEATURES

- Many types of histologic patterns have been reported; therefore, a drug etiology should always be in the differential diagnosis when evaluating a liver biopsy.
- Fulminant necrosis, zonal necrosis, prominent eosinophils, granulomas, and cholestatic hepatitis are suggestive of drug-related liver injury.
- Severe steatohepatitis mimicking alcoholic hepatitis: amiodarone, phenytoin (Figure 1-5D).
- Massive centrilobular necrosis: acetaminophen.

DIFFERENTIAL DIAGNOSIS

- Viral hepatitis
- Autoimmune hepatitis
- Ischemic necrosis

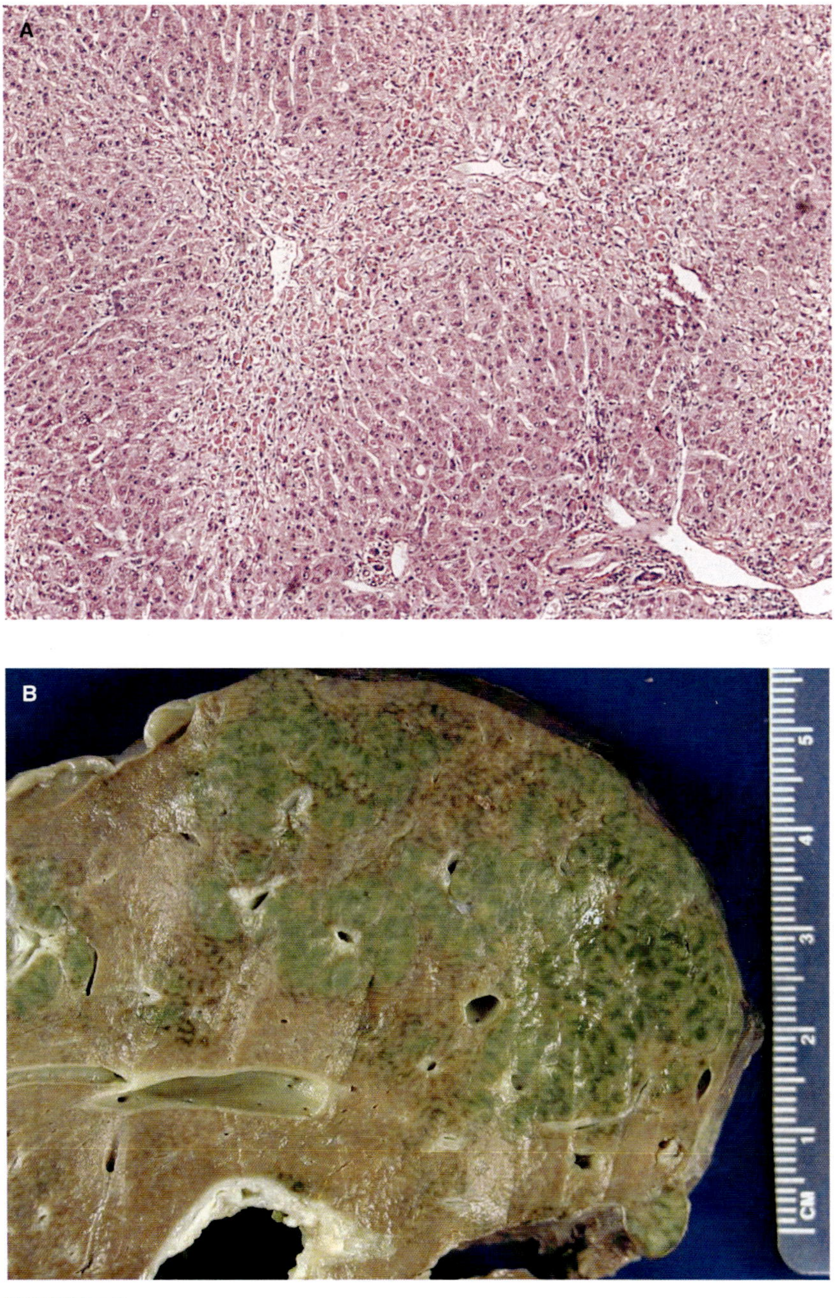

FIGURE 1-5

FIGURE 1-5 (A) Acetaminophen toxicity. Zone 3 necrosis without significant inflammation. Necrosis without inflammation is often seen with intrinsic toxins. This may be accompanied by marked steatosis in some cases. (B) Acute fulminant liver failure due to isoniazid required emergency transplantation.

(continued)

Drug-Induced Hepatic Necrosis *(continued)*

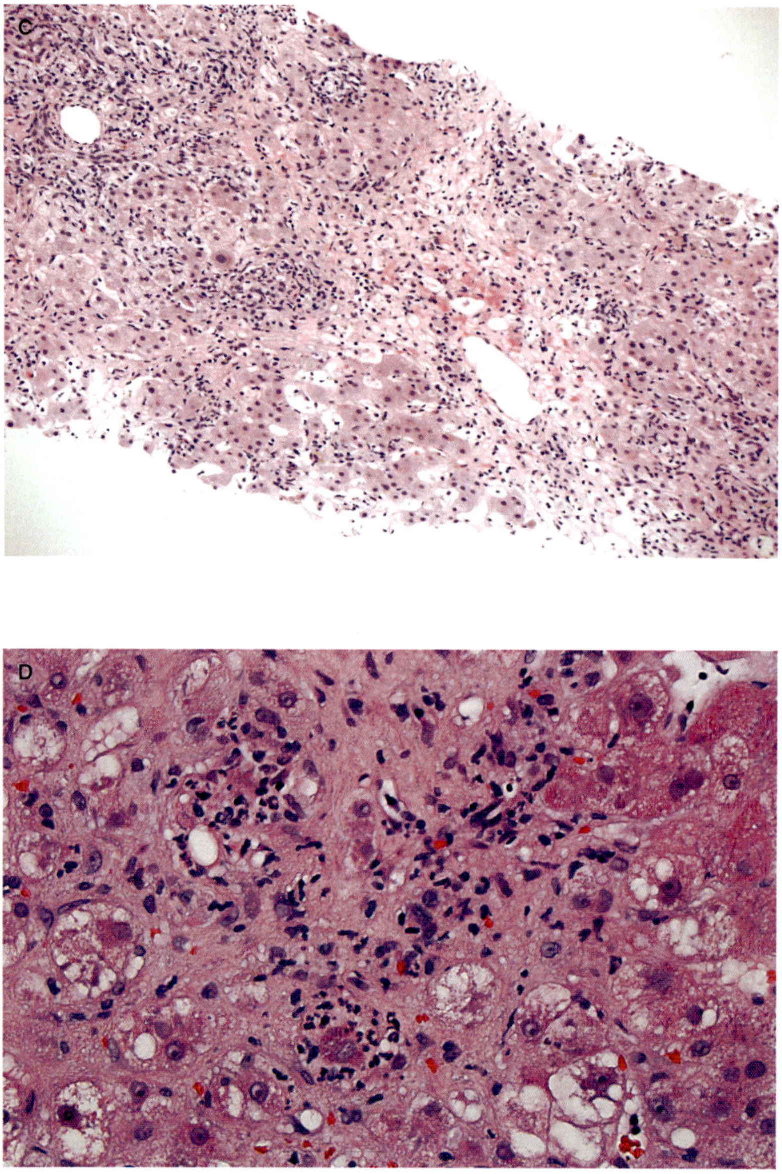

FIGURE 1-5

FIGURE 1-5 (C) Isoniazid-related acute hepatitis. Zone 3 necrosis with lymphoplasmacytic infiltrate is suggestive of drug-related liver injury. A necroinflammatory pattern is often seen with idiosyncratic toxins. (D) Ballooning degeneration and Mallory-Denk bodies due to amiodarone toxicity. Chronic changes such as prominent pericellular and centrilobular fibrosis are common as these occur in patients with heart failure with congestive fibrosis.

Pregnancy-Related Acute Hepatitis

DEFINITION

Acute liver diseases associated with pregnancy, including hyperemesis gravidarum, intrahepatic cholestasis of pregnancy, preeclampsia/eclampsia, hemolysis (H), elevated liver tests (EL) and low platelets (LP) and acute fatty liver of pregnancy. HELLP syndrome and acute fatty liver of pregnancy present with acute liver failure.

CLINICAL FEATURES

- About 2–12% of severe eclampsia cases complicated by HELLP syndrome.
- Both HELLP syndrome and acute fatty liver of pregnancy occur in the 3rd trimester.
- Early diagnosis and delivery critical.

HISTOLOGIC FEATURES

- HELLP syndrome: focal necrosis, periportal hemorrhage and fibrin deposits (Figure 1-6A).
- Acute fatty liver of pregnancy: severe microvesicular steatosis, hepatocellular swelling, and zone 3 perivenular canalicular cholestasis (Figure 1-6B).
- Oil red O stain sometimes required to confirm the diagnosis of acute fatty liver of pregnancy (Figure 1-6C).

DIFFERENTIAL DIAGNOSIS

- Liver diseases occurring coincidentally during pregnancy

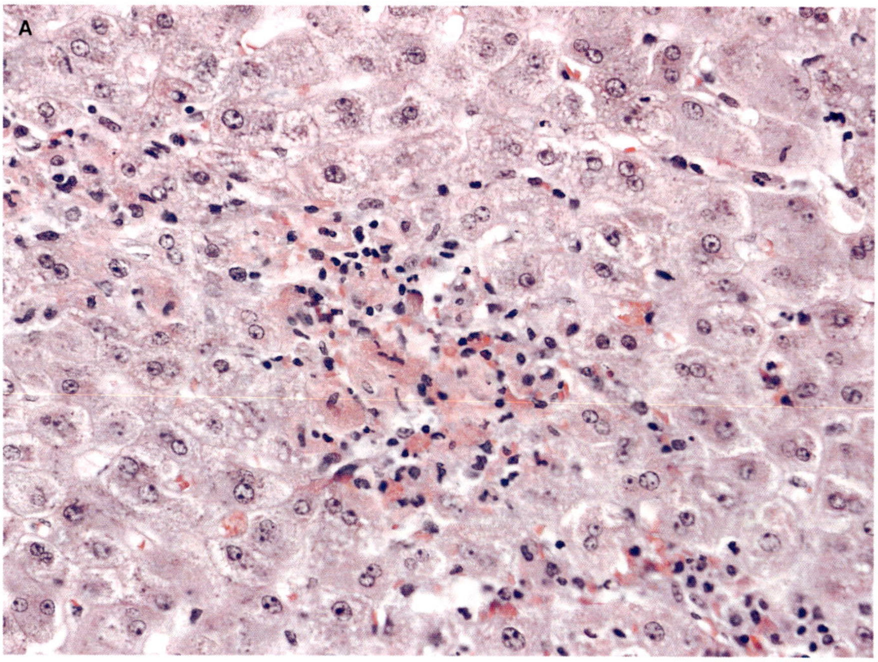

FIGURE 1-6

FIGURE 1-6 (A) HELLP syndrome: focal hepatocytic necrosis.

(continued)

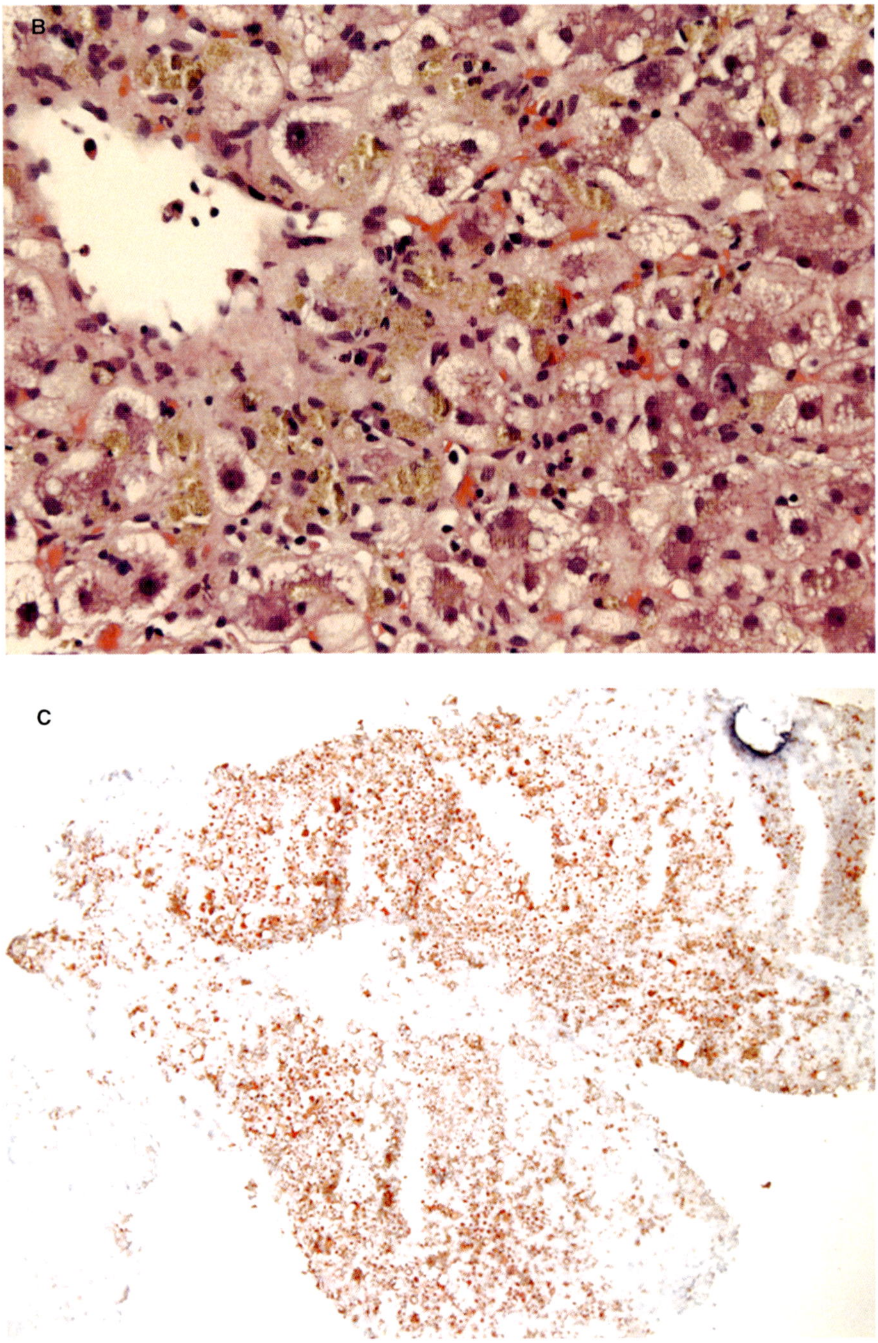

FIGURE 1-6

FIGURE 1-6 (B) Acute fatty liver of pregnancy. Hepatocytes with microvesicular steatosis and cholestasis. (C) Oil red O stain highlighting extensive microvesicular steatosis.

Chronic Hepatitis

2

CHRONIC VIRAL HEPATITIS

GRANULOMATOUS HEPATITIS

AUTOIMMUNE HEPATITIS

WILSON'S DISEASE

DRUG-INDUCED HEPATITIS

PARASITIC INFESTATION

Chronic Viral Hepatitis

DEFINITION

Persistent infections by a hepatotropic virus leading to chronic inflammation, hepatocyte injury and progressive fibrosis. Evidence of infection for more than 6 months is defined as chronic.

CLINICAL FEATURES

- General malaise; symptoms and signs of cirrhosis at later stage
- Diagnosis confirmed by serologic and/or molecular tests
- Liver biopsy helpful in predicting prognosis and monitoring therapy by assessment of the degree of necroinflammatory activity (grading) and fibrosis (staging)
- Biopsies also helpful in identifying a superimposed secondary disorder (e.g., nonalcoholic or alcoholic steatohepatitis)

PATHOLOGIC FEATURES

- Chronic hepatitis C: portal infiltration by lymphocytes and other inflammatory cells, with lymphoid aggregates (Figure 2-1A) and interface activity; mild lobular inflammation with spotty necrosis (acidophil bodies) (Figure 2-1B). Necroinflammation usually unevenly distributed.
- Chronic hepatitis B: ground-glass hepatocytes, due to accumulation of hepatitis B surface antigen in the endoplasmic reticulum of the hepatocytes; portal inflammation. Necroinflammation is diffuse (involving all areas evenly) (Figures 2-1C, D).
- Various grading and staging systems are available (the Knodell histology activity index [HAI] score, the Ishak-modified HAI score, the Metavir system, the Scheuer system, the Ludwig-Batt scheme, and so on).
- The algorithm commonly used for **needle biopsy** is outlined below:

GRADING OF DISEASE ACTIVITY

Grade 0 (No activity): essentially indistinguishable from normal liver; no interface activity

Grade 1 (Minimal activity): focal mild portal inflammation with scant interface activity; no significant lobular activity (one or two acidophil bodies are allowed)

Grade 2 (Mild activity): inflammatory infiltration involving less than 50% of portal tracts and/or interface activity seen at more than two foci, or scattered acidophil bodies easily identifiable (lobular activity)

Grade 3 (Moderate activity): inflammatory infiltration involving more than 50% of portal tracts, with moderate interface activity; and/or frequent lobular spotty necrosis (acidophil bodies)

Grade 4 (Severe activity): brisk interface activity (most of the portal tracts involved), and/or areas of confluent necrosis

STAGING OF FIBROSIS

Stage 0 (No significant fibrosis): indistinguishable from normal liver

Stage 1 (Mild portal fibrosis): fibrous portal expansion with occasional thread-like extension to periportal parenchyma or limiting plate (otherwise it would be nondistinguishable from normal as portal tracts vary in size)

Stage 2 (Periportal fibrosis): periportal extension involving more than 2 portal tracts, with rare portal-portal septa
Stage 3 (Septal/bridging fibrosis): evident fibrous septa connecting portal tracts
Stage 4 (Cirrhosis): cirrhosis

DIFFERENTIAL DIAGNOSIS

- Autoimmune hepatitis
- Drug-induced liver injury

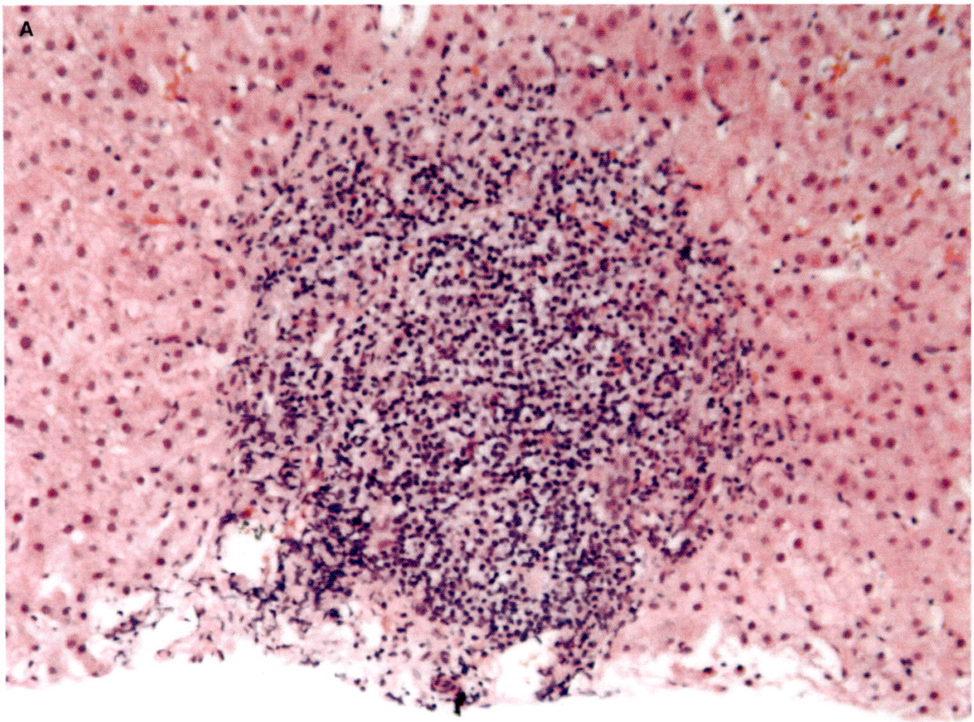

FIGURE 2-1

FIGURE 2-1 (A) Chronic hepatitis C. A lymphoid aggregate in a portal area. Lymphoid aggregates are not pathognomonic but are highly suggestive of hepatitis C.

(continued)

Chronic Viral Hepatitis *(continued)*

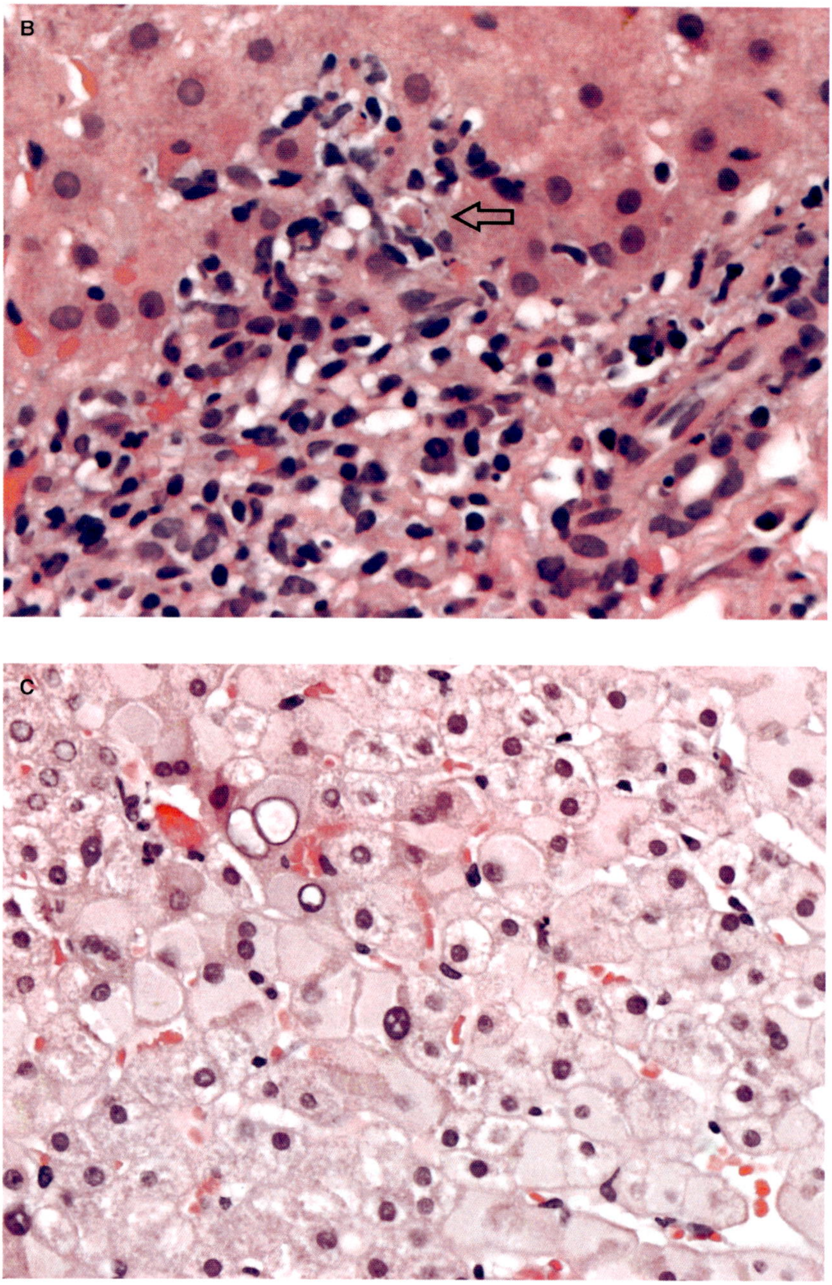

FIGURE 2-1

FIGURE 2-1 (B) Chronic hepatitis C. Interface activity (piecemeal necrosis; arrow: an acidophil body). (C) Chronic hepatitis B with ground-glass hepatocytes. Glassy eosinophilic cytoplasm represents endoplasmic reticulum with hepatitis B antigen. The inclusion pushes the cytoplasmic contents and the nuclei eccentrically.

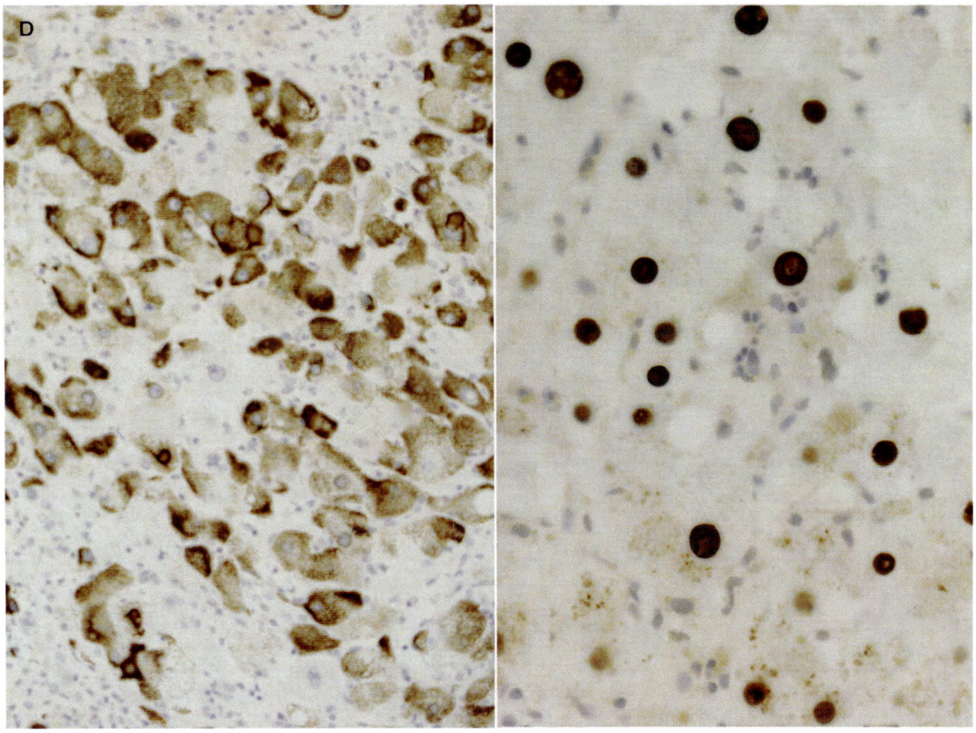

FIGURE 2-1

FIGURE 2-1 (D) Immunohistochemical staining for hepatitis B surface antigen (HBsAg, left) highlighting ground-glass hepatocytes. Cytoplasmic staining is usually associated with relatively low viral replication. Immunohistochemical staining for core antigen (HBcAg) showing positive nuclei confirms the presence of infection and replication (right).

Granulomatous Hepatitis

DEFINITION

The strict definition of granulomatous hepatitis requires the exclusion of known etiologies. However, several entities that give rise to hepatic granulomas are outlined in this section.

CLINICAL FEATURES

- Etiologies of hepatic granulomas include sarcoidosis (Figures 2-2A, B), infection (tuberculosis (Figure 2-2C), *Mycobacterium avium intracellulare* (Figure 2-2D), histoplasmosis), drugs (allopurinol), neoplasm (Hodgkin's disease), primary biliary cirrhosis, extrahepatic inflammatory disease (inflammatory bowel disease) and foreign substance (mineral oil). Rarely, granulomas may occur in association with chronic hepatitis C.

HISTOLOGIC FEATURES

- Type and location of granulomas are helpful clues to identify the etiology.
- Type of granuloma: microgranuloma, lipogranuloma, fibrin-ring granuloma, caseating and noncaseating epithelioid granuloma
- Sarcoidosis is characterized by well-formed epithelioid granulomas; drug injury may show either well-formed or poorly formed granulomas.
- Granulomas of primary biliary cirrhosis are epithelioid and can be well-formed or ill-formed; some are directly involved in bile duct injury.
- Necrotizing granulomas almost always indicate an infectious etiology.
- Fibrin ring granulomas have a distinctive appearance with central round clear space surrounded by an eosinophilic ring of fibrin that is highlighted by the Masson trichrome stain; they are usually associated with Q fever, caused by the rickettsia organism *Coxiella burnetii* (not specific).
- Microgranulomas and lipogranulomas are clusters of Kupffer cells or macrophages, which are nonspecific, and are usually seen in chronic hepatitis C or nonalcoholic steatohepatitis (NASH).

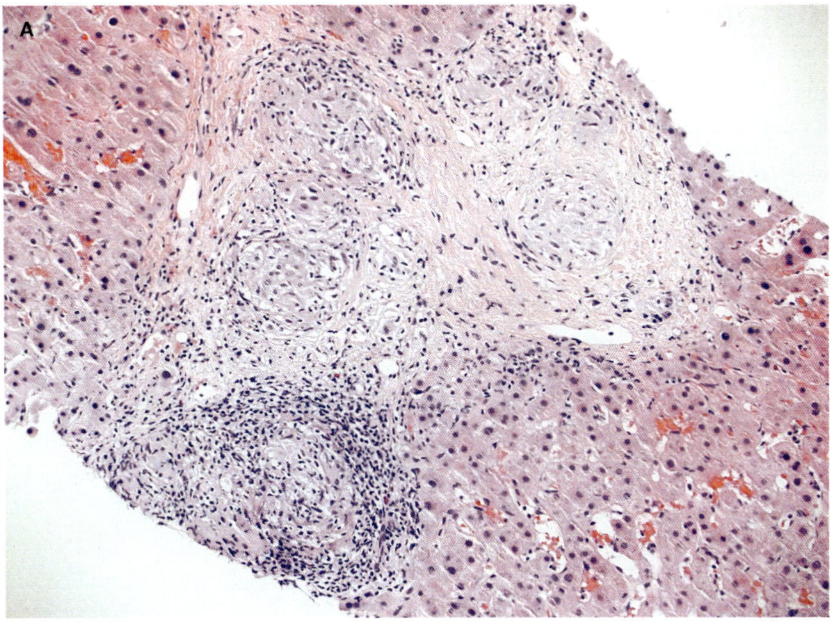

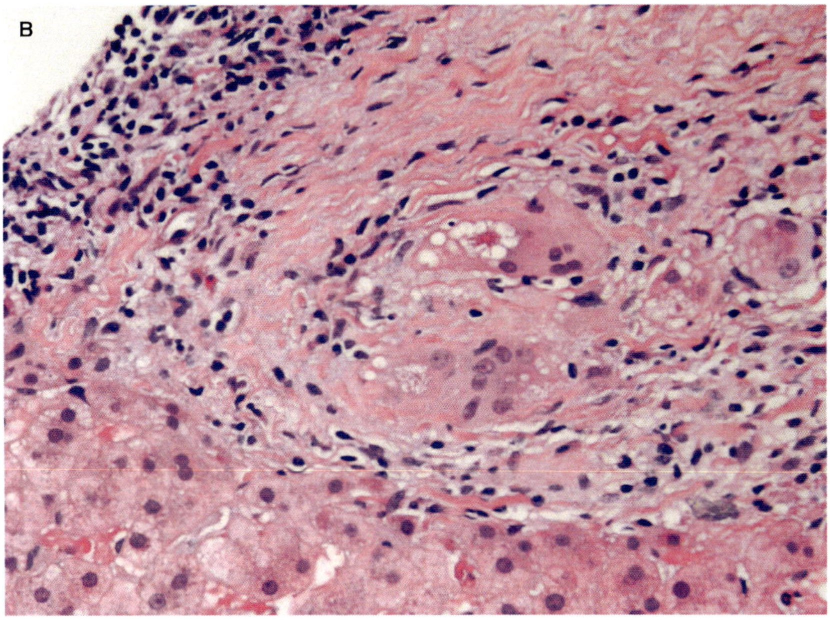

FIGURE 2-2

FIGURE 2-2 (A) Sarcoidosis with compact well-formed granuloma. Hyalinization is often seen. (B) Sarcoidosis with giant cell granuloma. The stellate-shaped asteroid body is usually found in the cytoplasm.

(continued)

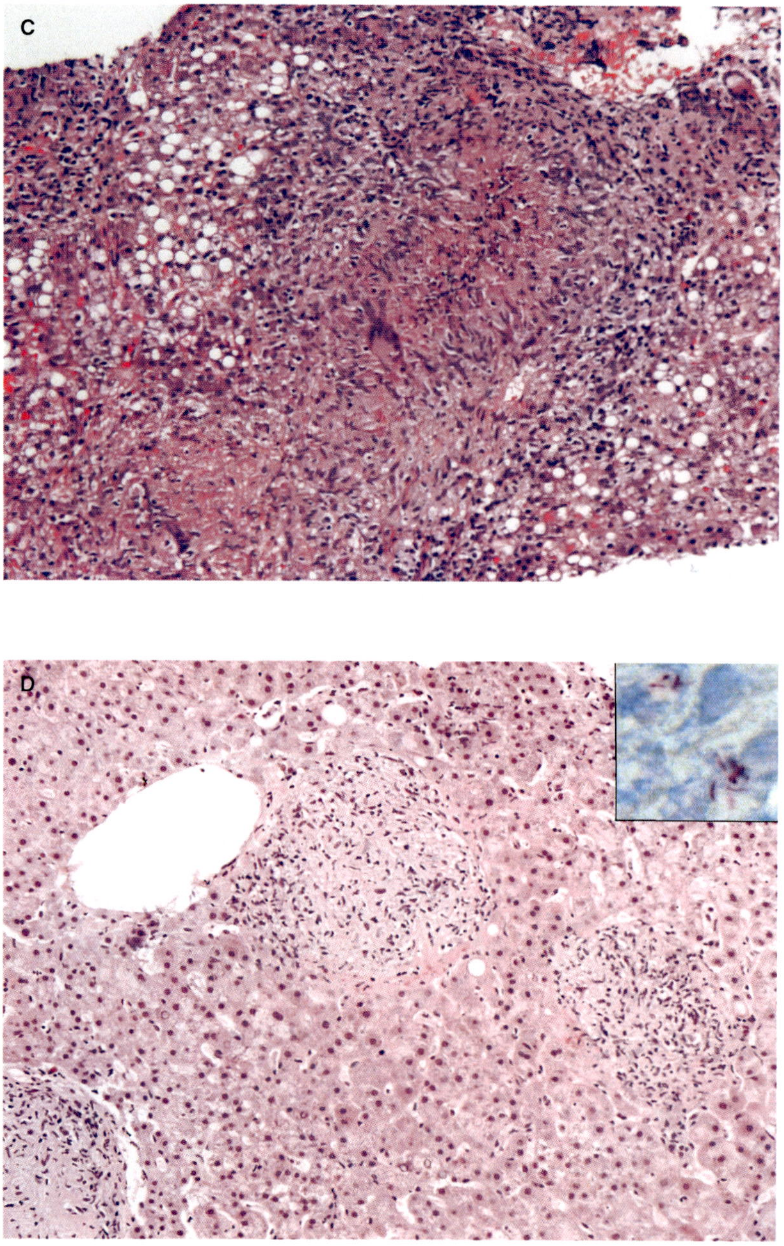

FIGURE 2-2

FIGURE 2-2 (C) Necrotizing granuloma with multinucleated giant cells due to disseminated tuberculosis. (D) Nonnecrotizing granuloma of *Mycobacterium avium-intracellulare* infection in a patient with human immunodeficiency virus infection. AFB stain shows organisms (insert).

Autoimmune Hepatitis

DEFINITION

Autoimmune hepatitis is an unresolving hepatitis associated with hypergammaglobulinemia and autoantibodies, which is responsive to immunosuppressive therapy.

CLINICAL FEATURES

- Diagnosis is based on a combination of clinical and laboratory features with exclusion of other chronic liver diseases.
- Antinuclear antibodies (ANA), anti-smooth muscle antibodies (SMA) and anti-liver-kidney microsomal (LKM) antibodies are the most commonly reported antibodies.
- Type 1: age at onset of bimodal distribution; ANA and/or SMA positive.
- Type 2: pediatric population; LKM positive; ANA and SMA negative.
- International autoimmune hepatitis group proposed a scoring system for the diagnosis. It evaluates 12 clinical comportments and is complex. Recently a simplified scoring system has been proposed. It evaluates only four clinical components.

HISTOLOGIC FEATURES

- Histology variable: interface hepatitis, lymphoplasmacytic infiltrate in portal tracts and extending into the lobules (Figure 2-3A), emperipolesis (engulfment of lymphocytes by hepatocytes) and hepatic rosette formation (Figure 2-3B).
- Acute fulminant form can occur (see Chapter 1).
- Presence of plasma cells in clusters at the area of interface activity favors autoimmune hepatitis over viral hepatitis.
- About one-third of autoimmune hepatitis cases have few or no plasma cells.
- Prominent mononuclear inflammation and hepatocyte dropout around a terminal hepatic venule may be seen in early phase (Figure 2-3C).
- Treated disease may present with normal histology or mild nonspecific chronic hepatitis.

DIFFERENTIAL DIAGNOSIS

- Viral hepatitis
- Drug-induced liver injury

(*continued*)

Autoimmune Hepatitis *(continued)*

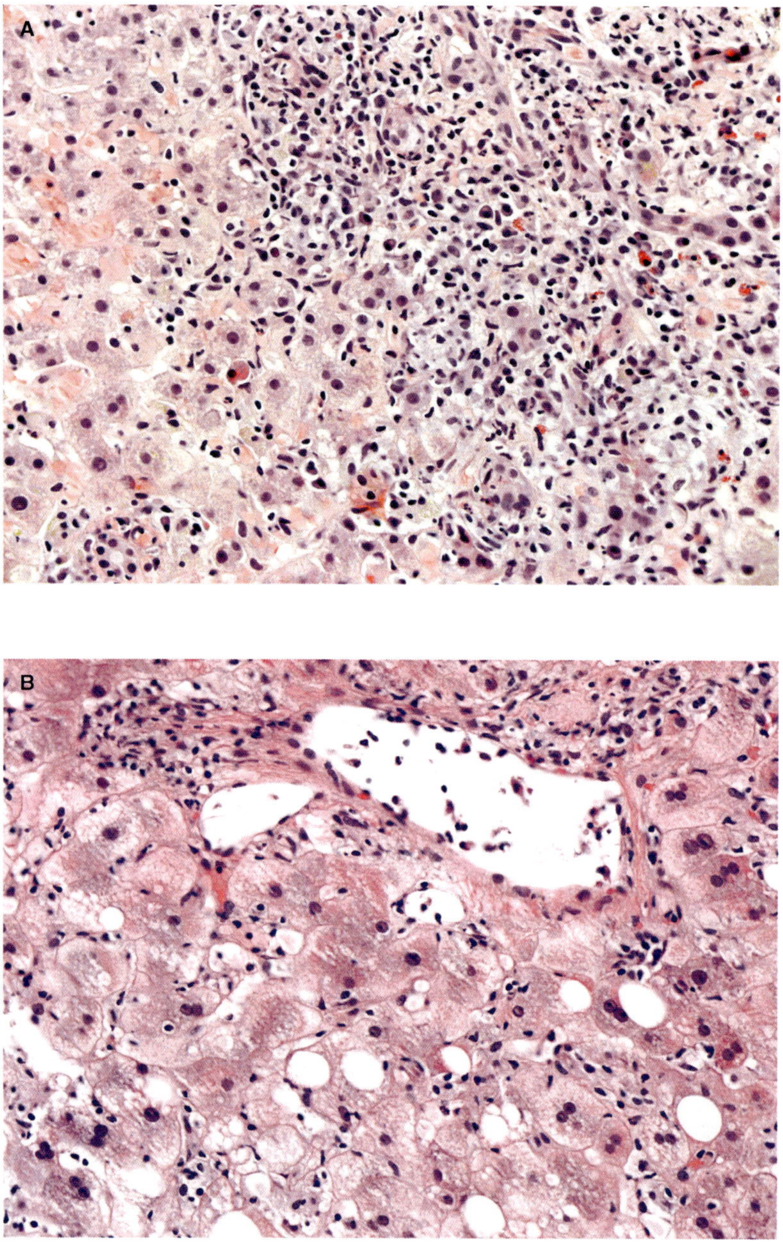

FIGURE 2-3

FIGURE 2-3 (A) Autoimmune hepatitis with interface activity. Portal lymphoplasmacytic infiltrate extending into the lobules with hepatocyte necrosis. (B) Autoimmune hepatitis. Hepatocyte ballooning degeneration, syncytial multinucleated giant cells, and rosettes formation are present. Engulfment of lymphocytes by hepatocytes (emperipolesis) is also noted.

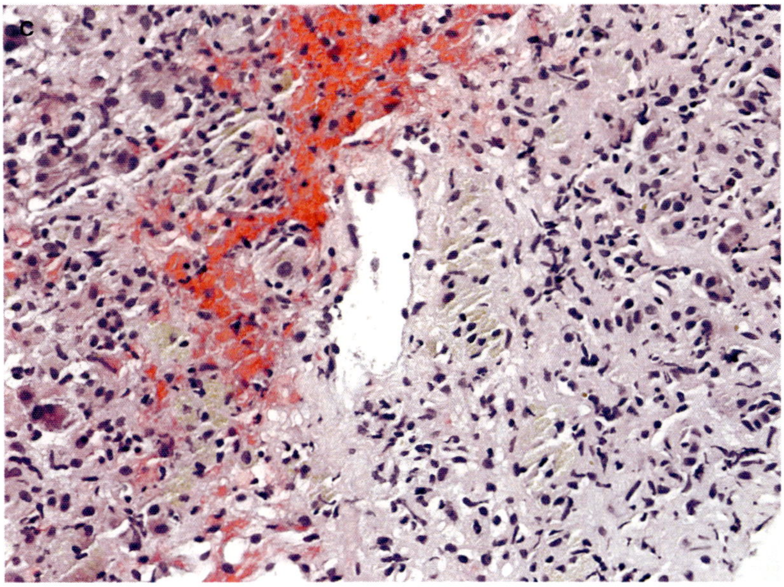

FIGURE 2-3

FIGURE 2-3 (C) Prominent mononuclear inflammation and hepatocyte dropout around a terminal hepatic venule may be seen in the active phase.

Wilson's Disease

DEFINITION

An autosomal recessive genetic disease with mutation of the ATP7B gene, which encodes for copper-dependent P-type ATPase (involved in copper transportation). Symptoms and signs are results of copper overload in various organs.

CLINICAL FEATURES

- Wilson's disease should be considered in any individual with liver abnormality of uncertain cause and neurologic disorder.
- Assessment should include clinical history, physical examination (Kayser-Fleischer rings), liver function tests, hematology (for hemolysis), serum copper, and ceruloplasmin and 24-hour urinary copper excretion.

HISTOLOGIC FEATURES

- Chronic hepatitis (mononuclear portal inflammation, interface activity and fibrosis) (Figure 2-4A).
- Steatosis, Mallory-Denk body, and glycogenated nuclei.
- Fulminant cases show parenchymal necrosis.
- Rhodamine stain may show increased copper stain in zone 1 hepatocytes, but can be negative (Figure 2-4B).
- Liver biopsy quantitative copper concentrations remain the best biochemical evidence for Wilson's disease.

DIFFERENTIAL DIAGNOSIS

- NASH
- Other chronic hepatitis, such as autoimmune hepatitis

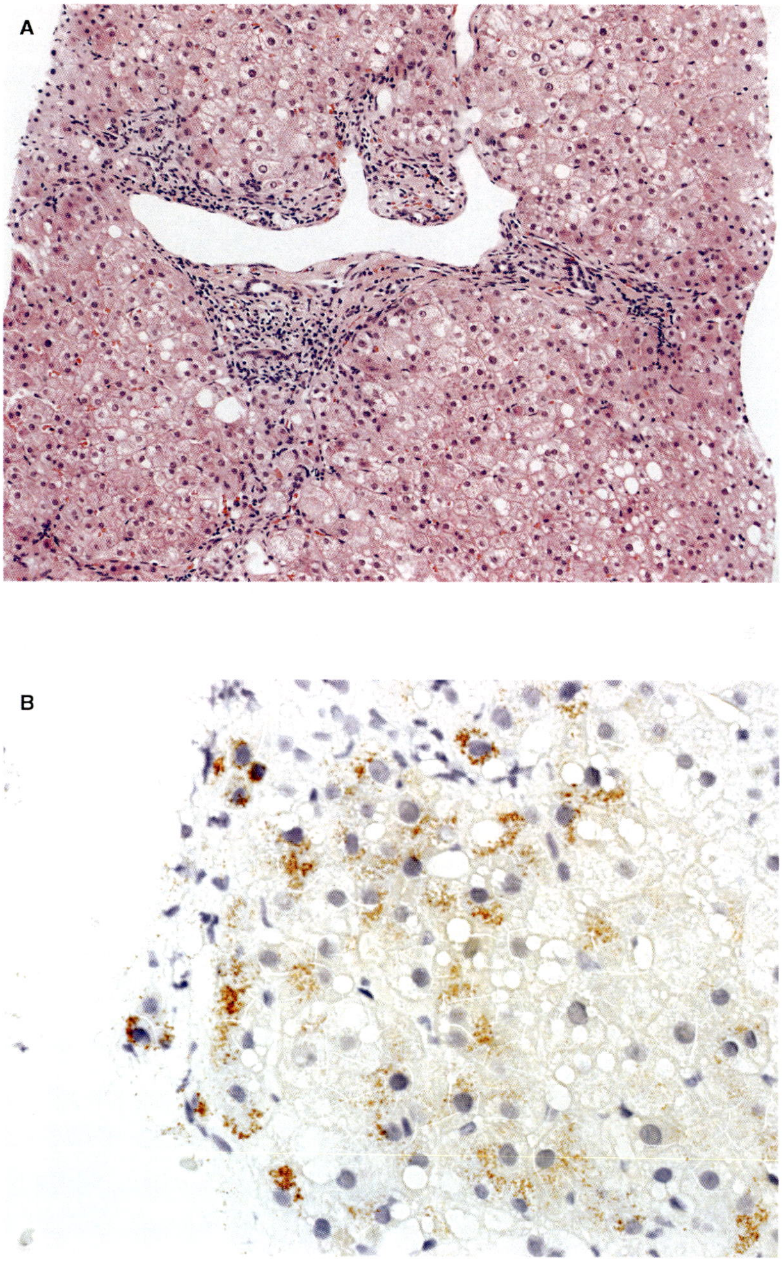

FIGURE 2-4

FIGURE 2-4 (A) Wilson's disease. Portal inflammatory infiltration, with mild steatosis. (B) Rhodamine stain showing increased copper deposits in periportal (zone 1) hepatocytes.

Drug-Induced Hepatitis

DEFINITION

Abnormality of liver biochemical test related to intake of drug and toxin. Many drugs are known to cause hepatic injury resembling chronic viral hepatitis or autoimmune hepatitis.

CLINICAL FEATURES (SEE CHAPTER 1)

- Cholestatic hepatitis (combined hepatocellular–cholestatic injury) is the most common form of drug-induced liver injury (Figures 2-5A, B).
- Some drug (minocycline, nitrofurantoin, statin) may cause autoimmune hepatitis-like injury with positive antinuclear or anti-smooth muscle antibodies and hyperglobulinemia (Figure 2-5C).

HISTOLOGIC FEATURES

- Chronic hepatitis pattern is characterized by mixed portal inflammation.
- Some drugs (amiodarone, methotrexate) may cause fibrosis and cirrhosis.
- Cholestasis in a background of chronic hepatitis
- Cholestatic injury with inflammation: allopurinol, cimetidine, ibuprofen, antibiotics such as amoxicillin-clavulanate, carbamazepine, nitrofurantoin; without inflammation: anabolic steroid, estrogen, phenytoin.
- Bile duct injury, ductopenia, or cholangitis may be seen.

DIFFERENTIAL DIAGNOSIS

- Viral hepatitis
- Autoimmune hepatitis
- Wilson's disease

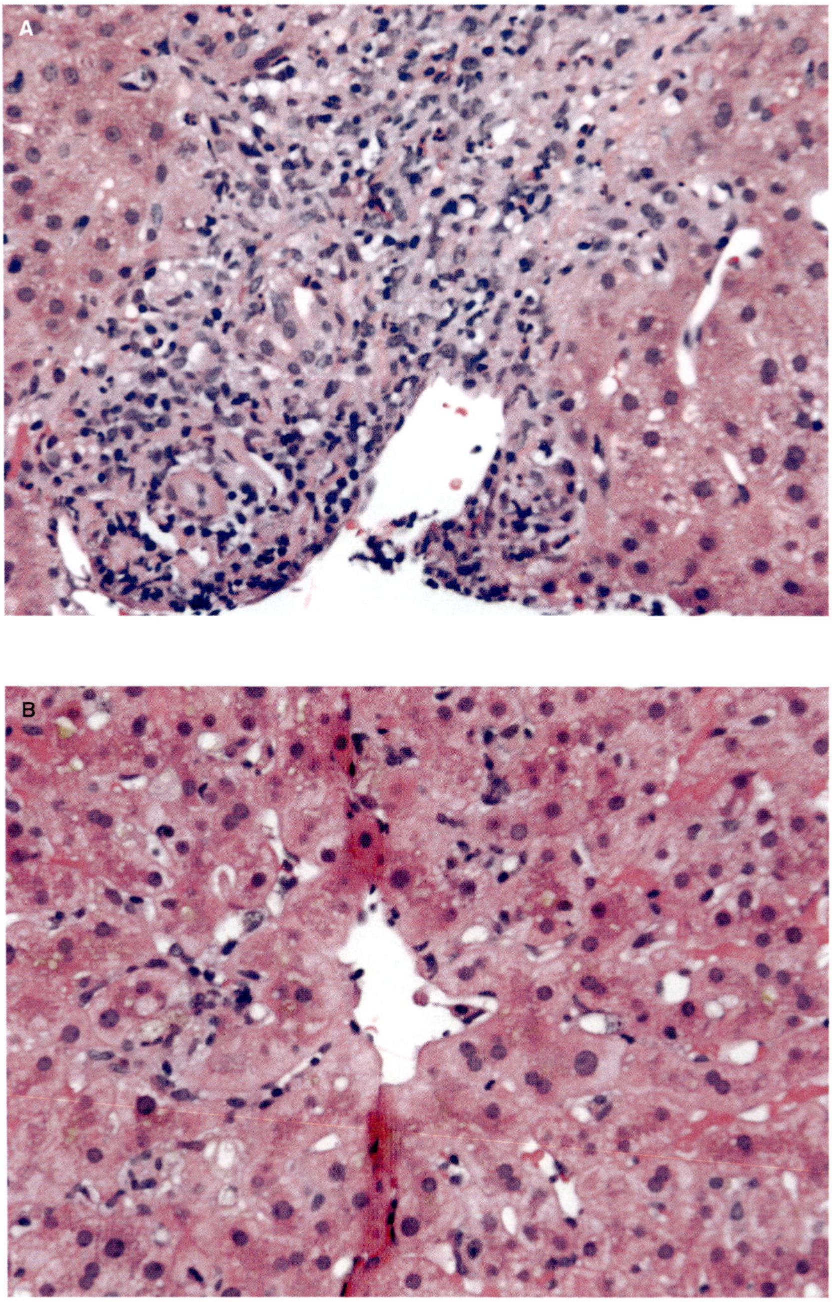

FIGURE 2-5

FIGURE 2-5 (A) Amoxicillin-clavulanate-related liver injury. Bile duct injury associated with mixed portal chronic inflammation, lymphocytes predominant, mixed with plasma cells, eosinophils and neutrophils. (B) Cholestasis in zone 3.

(*continued*)

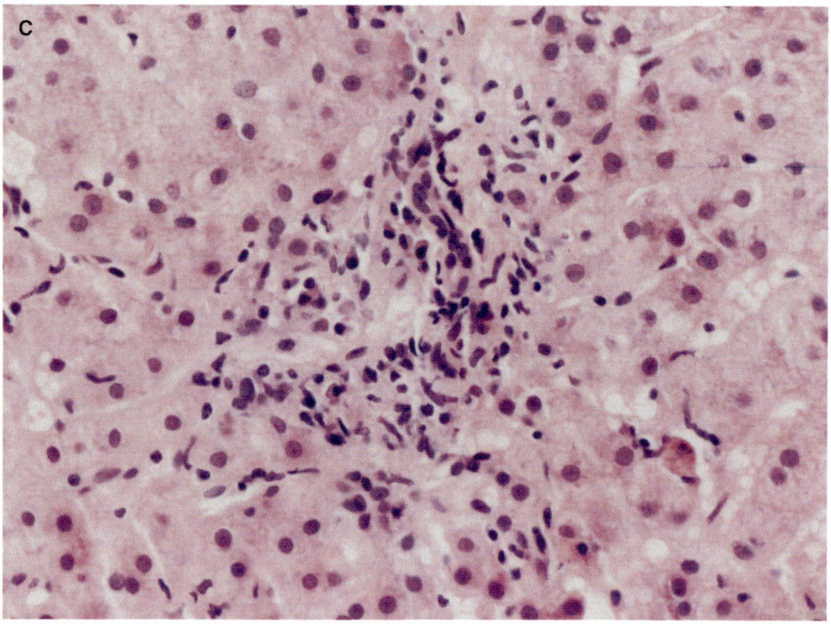

FIGURE 2-5

FIGURE 2-5 (C) Minocycline-related liver injury. Lymphoplasmacytic portal inflammation is evident.

Parasitic Infestation

DEFINITION

Hepatic dysfunction caused by parasites.

CLINICAL FEATURES

SCHISTOSOMIASIS

- A major tropical disease that causes portal hypertension worldwide
- *Schistosoma mansoni* found in Latin America, Africa, and the Middle East
- *Schistosoma japonicum* found in Southeast Asia

ECHINOCOCCOSIS

- Echinococcosis widely distributed worldwide

PATHOLOGIC FEATURES

SCHISTOSOMIASIS

- In early acute phase, ova appear within the portal tracts and form eosinophilic granulomas (Figures 2-6A, B).
- Symmer's pipe stem fibrosis: peri-granulomatous fibrous reaction, periportal fibrosis develops and occludes the portal vein leading to portal hypertension without cirrhosis.
- The eggs degenerate and die, becoming empty shells that often calcify.

ECHINOCOCCOSIS (HYDATID CYST)

- Unilocular cysts related to Echinococcosis *granulosus*, and composed of an external acellular membrane, middle laminated layer, and inner germinal layer (Figures 2-6C, D)
- Multilocular cysts related to Echinococcosis *multilocularis*, and less common

DIFFERENTIAL DIAGNOSIS

- Granulomatous hepatitis for Schistosomiasis
- Amebic abscess for Echinococcosis

(*continued*)

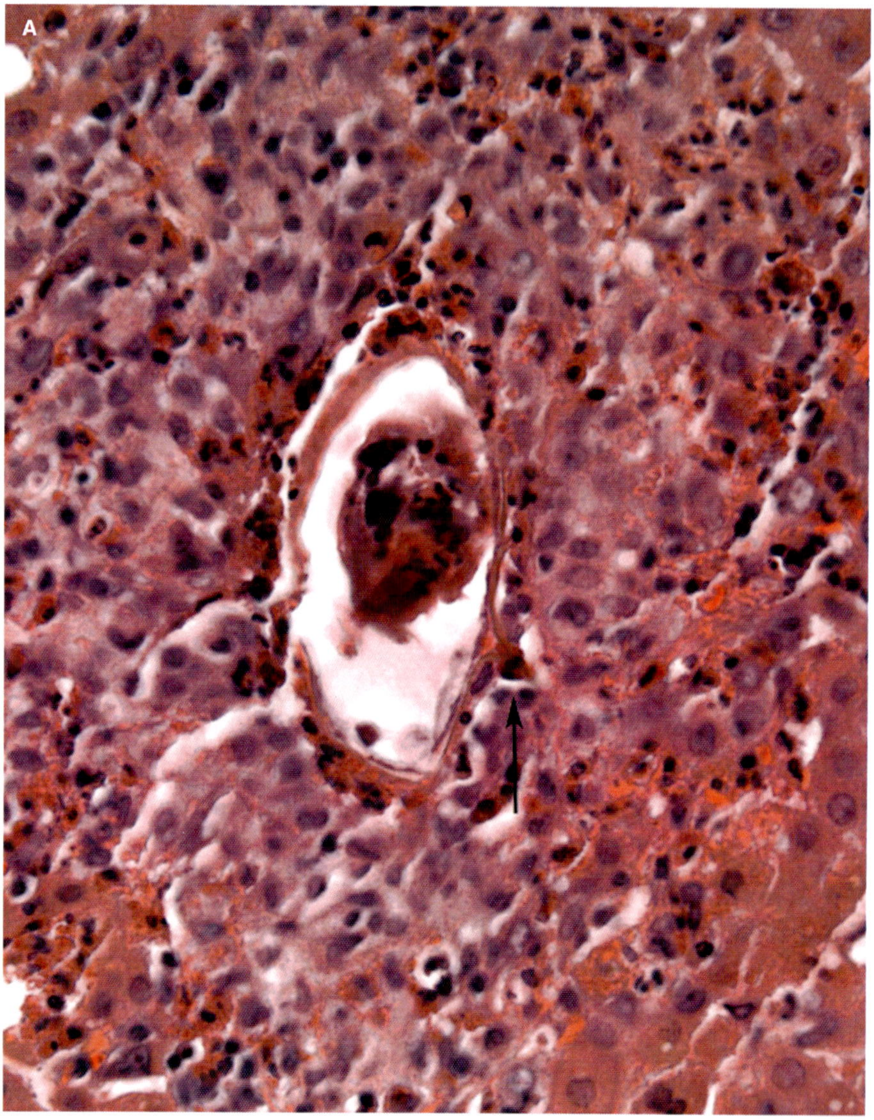

FIGURE 2-6

FIGURE 2-6 (A) *Schistosomiasis mansoni*. An eosinophilic granuloma containing an ovum with lateral spine (arrow).

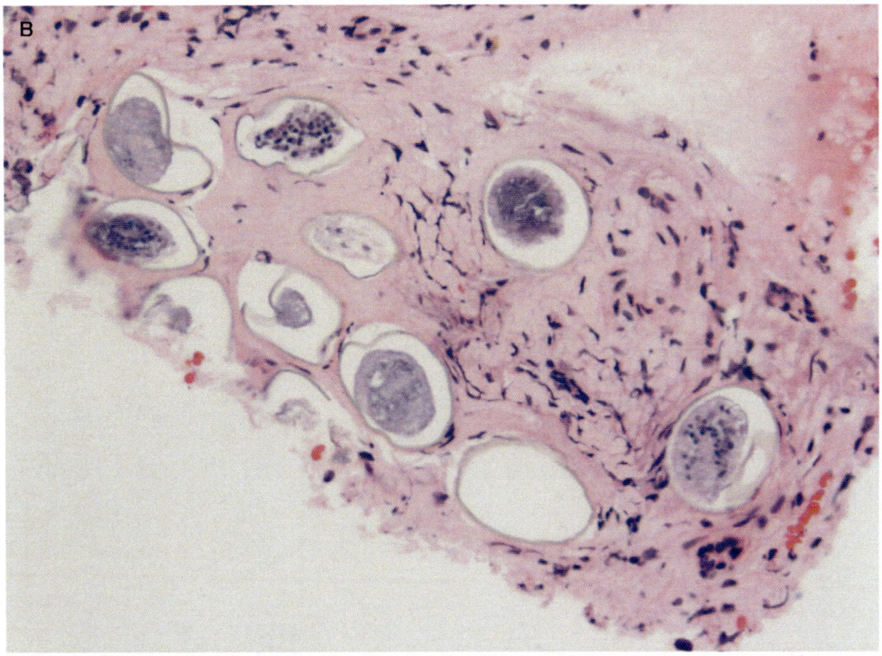

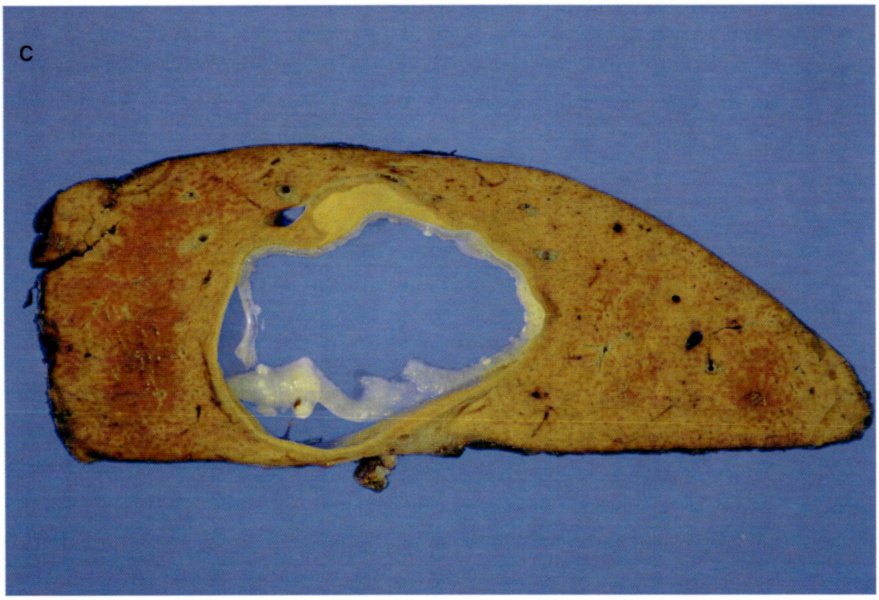

FIGURE 2-6

FIGURE 2-6 (B) *Schistosomiasis japonica*. Numerous dead ova within fibrotic portal tracts. *Schistosomiasis japonica* is smaller than *mansoni*. (C) Gross photo of a hydatid cyst.

(*continued*)

Parasitic Infestation *(continued)*

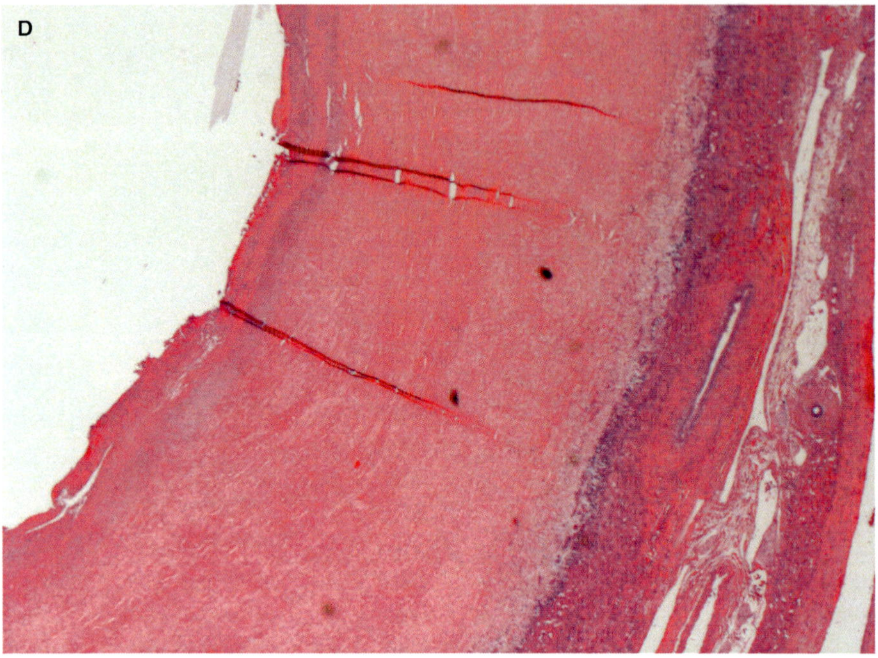

FIGURE 2-6

FIGURE 2-6 (D) Echinococcosis (hydatid cyst). The cyst wall is composed of acellular hyalinized fibrous tissue.

Biliary Diseases and Cholestasis

3

BILIARY OBSTRUCTION AND ASCENDING CHOLANGITIS

LIVER INVOLVEMENT IN SEPSIS

PRIMARY BILIARY CIRRHOSIS (PBC)

PRIMARY SCLEROSING CHOLANGITIS

OVERLAP SYNDROME

Biliary Obstruction and Ascending Cholangitis

DEFINITION
Mechanical obstruction of extrahepatic or large intrahepatic bile ducts. Etiologies include stones; neoplasms of the extrahepatic biliary tree, ampulla of Vater or head of the pancreas; primary or secondary sclerosing cholangitis; and biliary atresia.

CLINICAL FEATURES
- Abdominal pain, jaundice, steatorrhea, and pruritus
- Complications include bacterial cholangitis and cirrhosis
- Elevated bilirubin and alkaline phosphatase

HISTOLOGIC FEATURES
- Centrilobular hepatocellular and canalicular cholestasis (Figure 3-1A)
- Bile ductular reaction (proliferating ductules with an associated mixed inflammatory cellular infiltrate) and edema in portal tracts (Figures 3-1B, C)
- Bile plugs in bile ducts, or bile lakes (late)
- Neutrophilic infiltrate around bile ducts
- Ascending cholangitis: neutrophilic infiltration of ductal epithelium and/or lumen
- Cholate stasis (feathery degeneration), characterized by swollen hepatocytes due to toxic effect of bile acids or bile salts (Figure 3-1D)
- Ill-formed Mallory-Denk bodies; increased copper and copper-binding protein in periportal hepatocytes in chronic cholestasis
- Cirrhosis due to cholestatic disease characterized by irregular regenerative nodules (jigsaw puzzle pattern)

DIFFERENTIAL DIAGNOSIS
- Sepsis
- Drug-induced liver injury

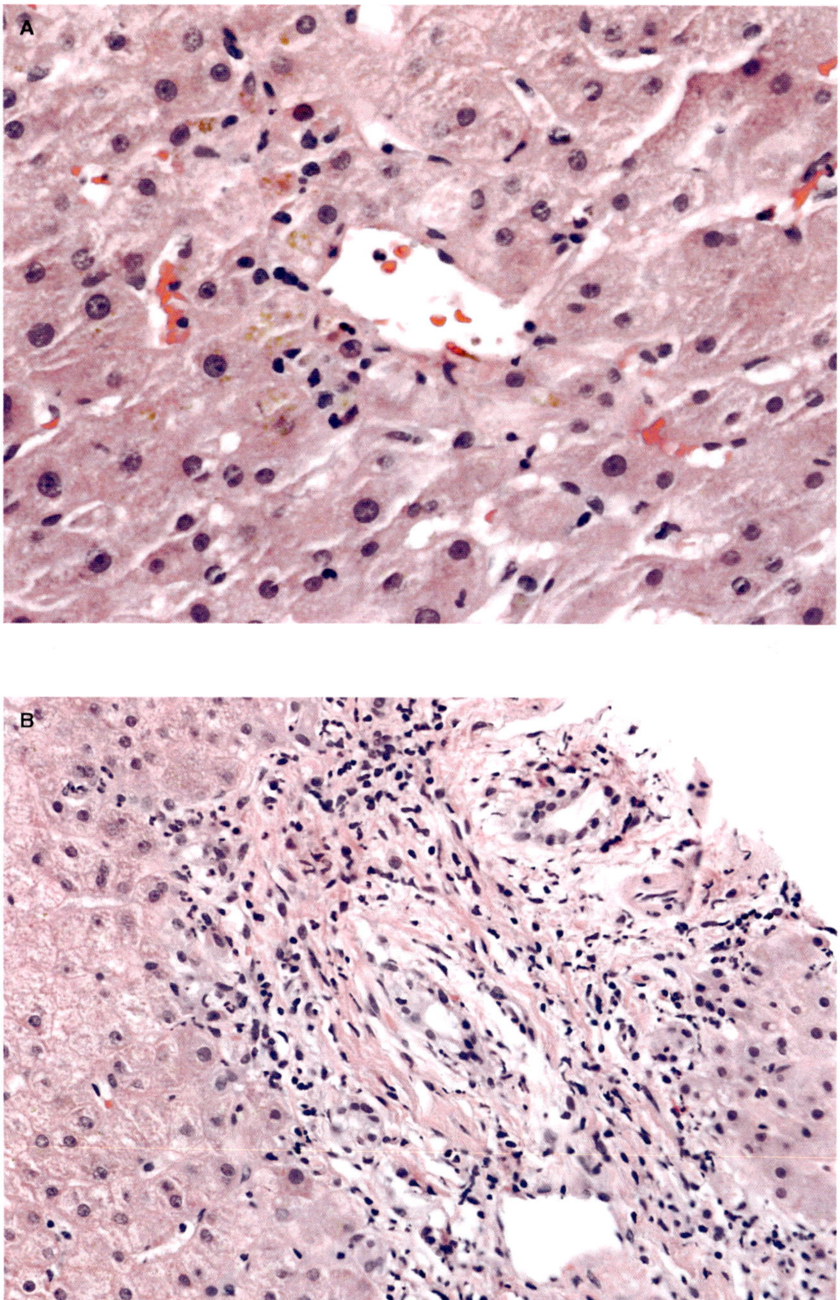

FIGURE 3-1

FIGURE 3-1 (A) Cholestasis present in zone 3 hepatocytes (hepatocellular cholestasis). (B) Early stage of biliary obstruction: periductal edema and mixed inflammatory cellular infiltration.

(continued)

Biliary Obstruction and Ascending Cholangitis *(continued)*

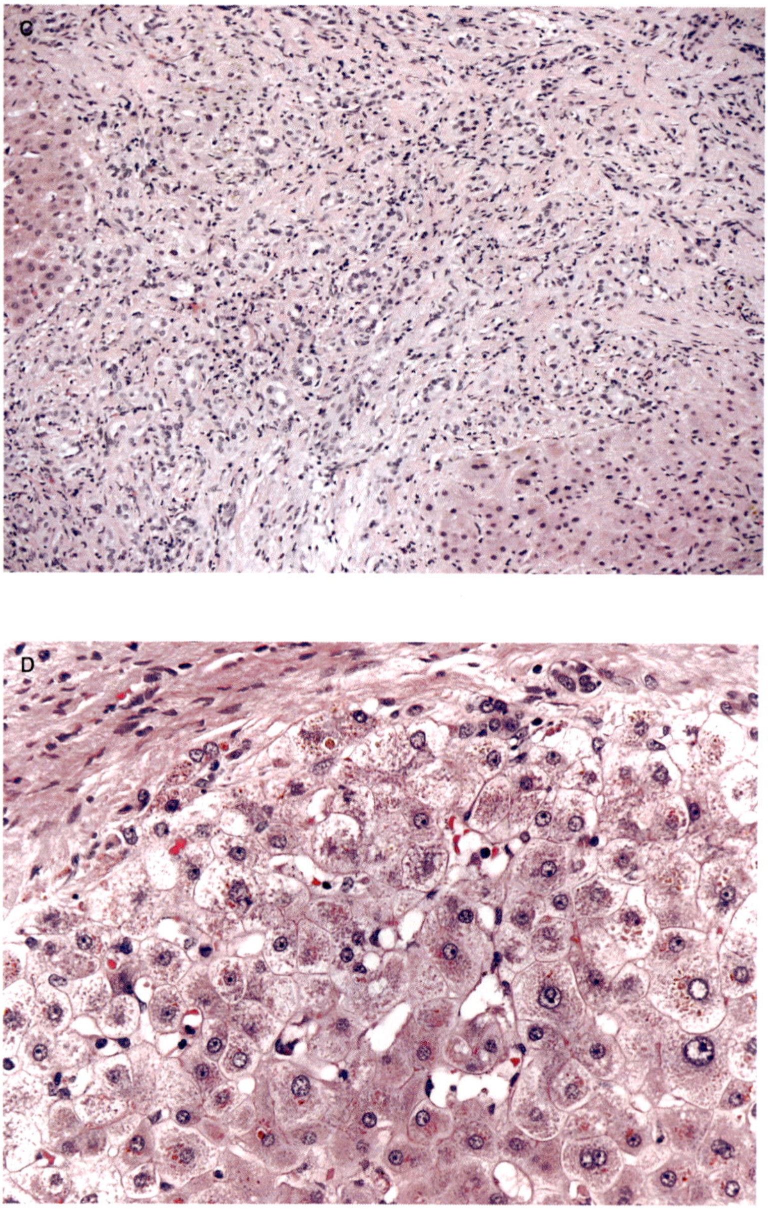

FIGURE 3-1

FIGURE 3-1 (C) Late stage of biliary obstruction: ductular proliferation associated with periductal fibrosis. (D) Feathery degeneration characterized by swollen or ballooned hepatocytes impregnated with bilirubin in the periphery of a nodule (late stage).

Liver Involvement in Sepsis

DEFINITION

Hepatic injury seen in septicemia and severe bacterial infection

CLINICAL FEATURES

- Jaundice
- Etiologies include liver infection, extrahepatic infection or toxic shock syndrome, and any other cause of sepsis

HISTOLOGIC FEATURES

- Cholangitis lenta: biliary stasis or bile plugs in bile ductules at the periphery of portal tracts (canals of Hering) (Figure 3-2A)
- Neutrophilic infiltration around affected ductules (Figure 3-2B)
- Zone 3 canalicular cholestasis

DIFFERENTIAL DIAGNOSIS

- Large bile duct obstruction
- Drug-induced liver injury

(*continued*)

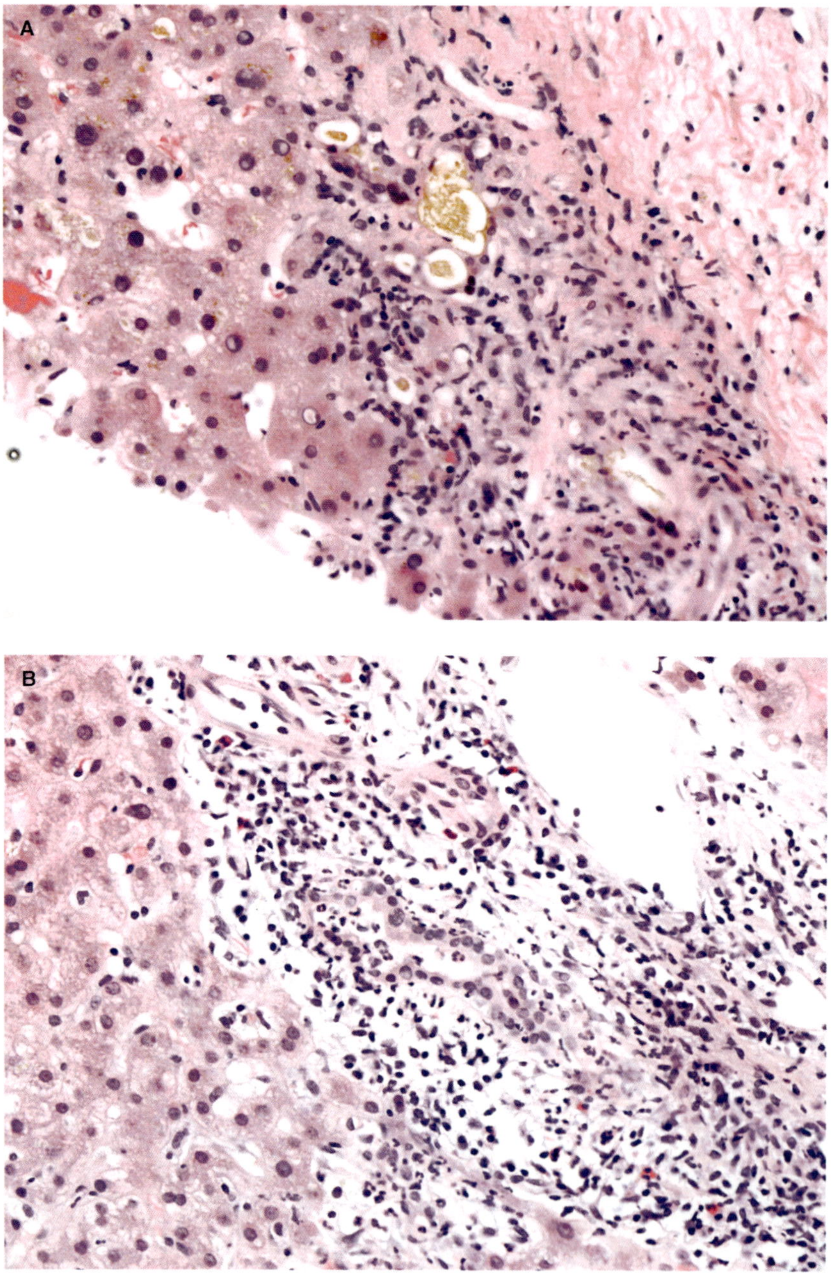

FIGURE 3-2

FIGURE 3-2 (A) Cholangitis lenta: bile ductules contain inspissated bile and portal tracts with mixed inflammatory infiltration. (B) Ascending cholangitis. Neutrophils are present in the lumen of bile ducts.

Primary Biliary Cirrhosis (PBC)

DEFINITION

An autoimmune disease primarily affecting the intrahepatic bile ducts and causing progressive destruction and loss of intrahepatic bile ducts

CLINICAL FEATURES

- Primarily affects middle-aged women
- Fatigue, abdominal pain, pruritus; jaundice in end-stage disease
- Persistent elevation of alkaline phosphatase, bilirubin and anti-mitochondrial antibodies (AMA)
- Autoimmune cholangitis: about 10% of cases are negative for AMA, half of which are positive for antinuclear antibodies and/or smooth muscle antibodies (SMA)

HISTOLOGIC FEATURES

- Florid bile duct lesion (nonsuppurative destructive cholangitis): lymphoplasmacytic inflammation, injury to bile duct epithelium (Figures 3-3A, B)
- Noncaseating granulomas
- Chronic cholestasis
- Increased copper accumulation in periportal hepatocytes
- Scheuer staging system
  - Stage 1: florid bile duct lesion
  - Stage 2: ductular proliferation
  - Stage 3: bile duct loss (Figure 3-3C)
  - Stage 4: cirrhosis (Figure 3-3D)

DIFFERENTIAL DIAGNOSIS

- Biliary obstruction
- Drug-induced liver injury
- Autoimmune hepatitis (AIH)
- Primary sclerosing cholangitis (PSC)

(*continued*)

Primary Biliary Cirrhosis (PBC) *(continued)*

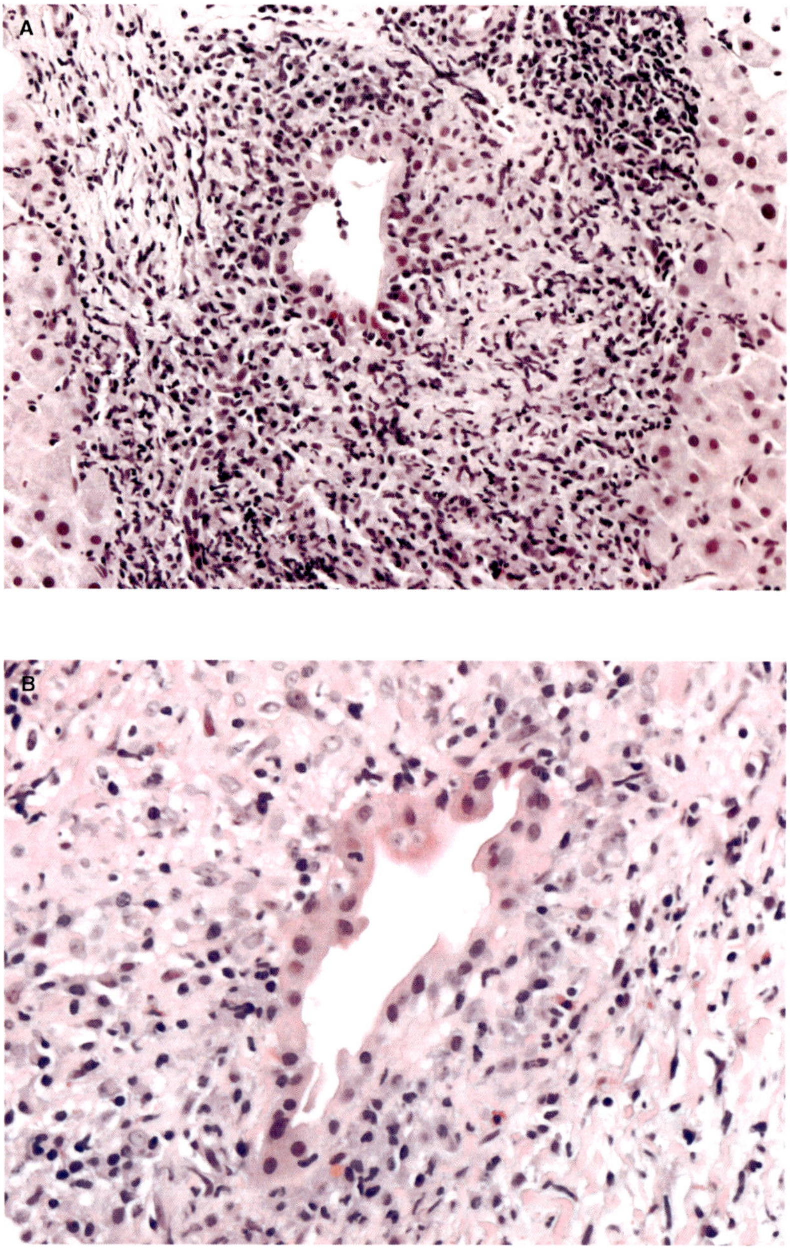

FIGURE 3-3

FIGURE 3-3 (A) Florid bile duct lesion with poorly formed granuloma. There is lymphoplasmacytic portal inflammation with minimal interface activity in the background. (B) Florid bile duct lesion. Bile duct injury characterized by eosinophilic epithelium, intraepithelial lymphocytes, and vacuolization of bile duct epithelium.

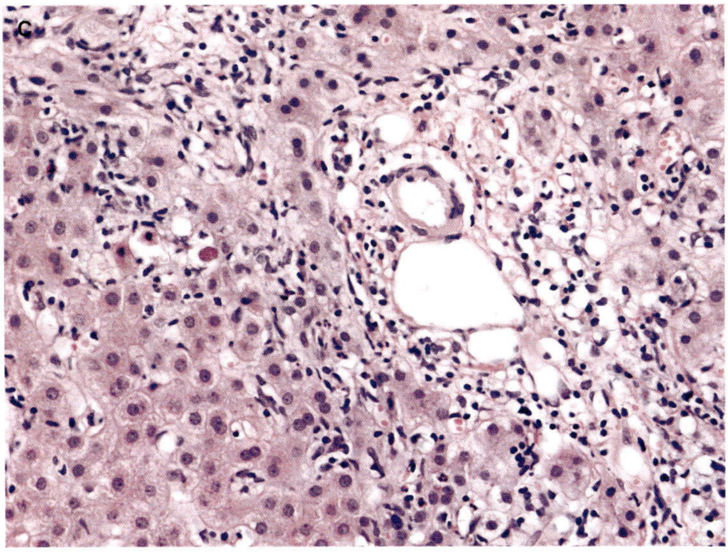

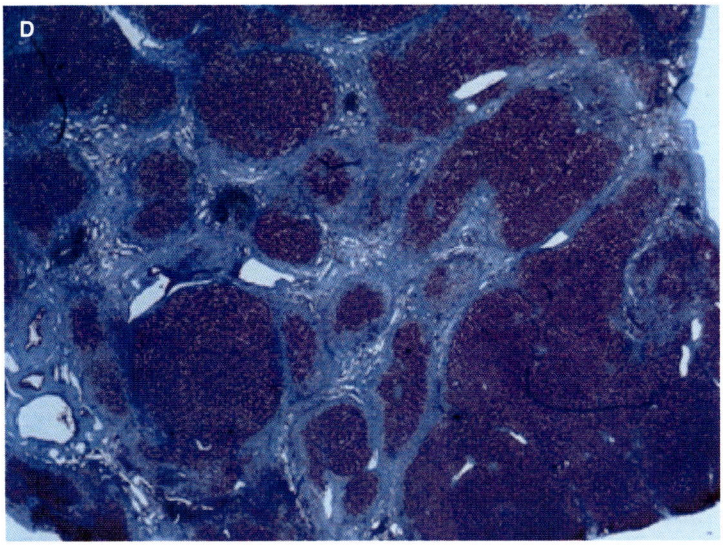

FIGURE 3-3

FIGURE 3-3 (C) Bile duct loss. In the portal triad, there is a hepatic artery and portal vein but no interlobular bile duct. (D) Biliary cirrhosis showing jigsaw puzzle pattern.

Primary Sclerosing Cholangitis

DEFINITION

Chronic autoimmune inflammation and sclerosis (periductal fibrosis) of the extrahepatic and intrahepatic bile ducts, leading to progressive fibrosis and cirrhosis

CLINICAL FEATURES

- Male predominance; usually diagnosed around 40 years of age, but affects all ages
- Strong association with inflammatory bowel disease: about 65% occur in patients with ulcerative colitis, 10% in Crohn's disease
- Pathogenesis: a combination of genetic predisposition and immune-mediated disorder
- Fatigue, pruritus
- "Beaded appearance" of the bile duct on cholangiography
- Increased risk of developing cholangiocarcinoma
- Overlaps with AIH, particularly among pediatric population
- No effective medical treatment; transplantation curative

HISTOLOGIC FEATURES

- Often nonspecific in liver biopsies, including changes related to bile duct stricture
- Classic histologic appearance of concentric periductal "onion skin" fibrosis in medium and large-size bile ducts (Figure 3-4A)
- Fibrous obliteration of bile ducts and ductopenia (Figures 3-4B, C)
- Chronic cholestasis
- Extrahepatic bile ducts may show ulceration, xanthogranulomatous inflammation, and fibrosis (Figure 3-4D)
- Biliary cirrhosis
- Small duct PSC: variant of PSC affecting only small intrahepatic bile ducts, with normal cholangiography

DIFFERENTIAL DIAGNOSIS

- Secondary sclerosing cholangitis
- Primary biliary cirrhosis

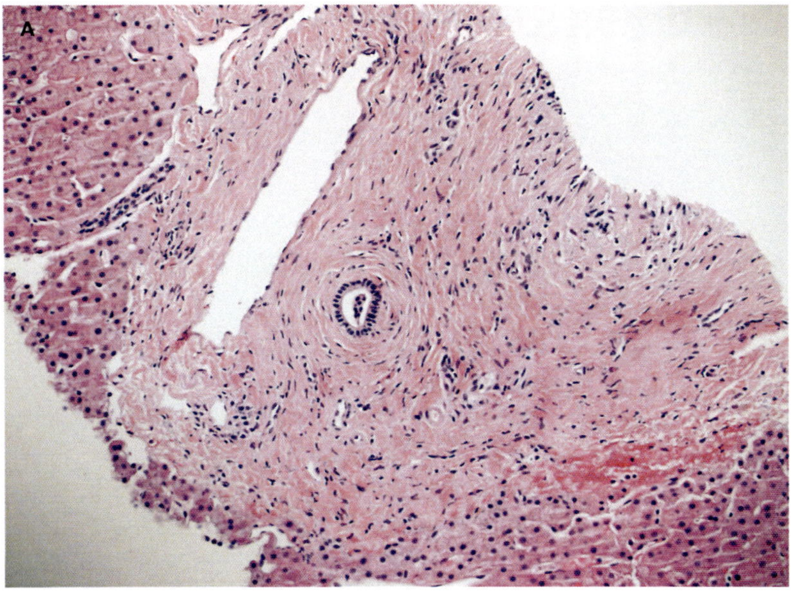

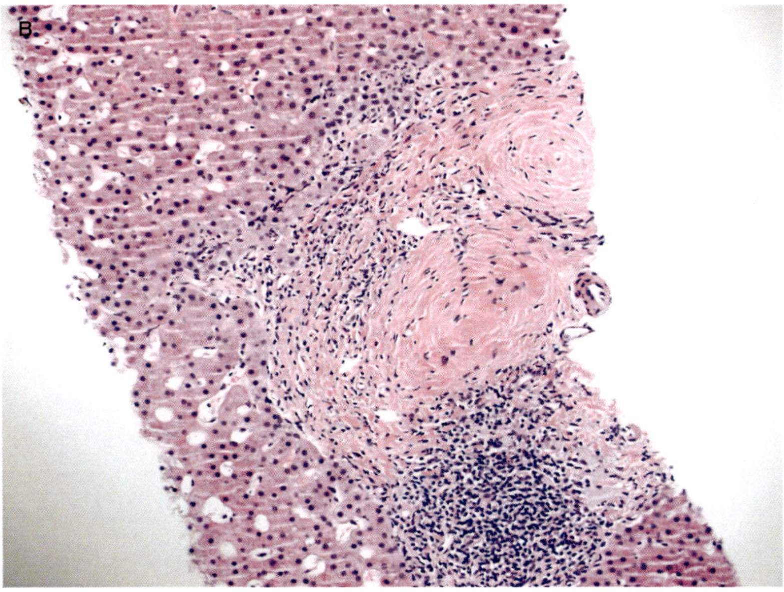

FIGURE 3-4

FIGURE 3-4 (A) Concentric onion skin periductal fibrosis. (B) Fibrous obliteration of bile duct.

(*continued*)

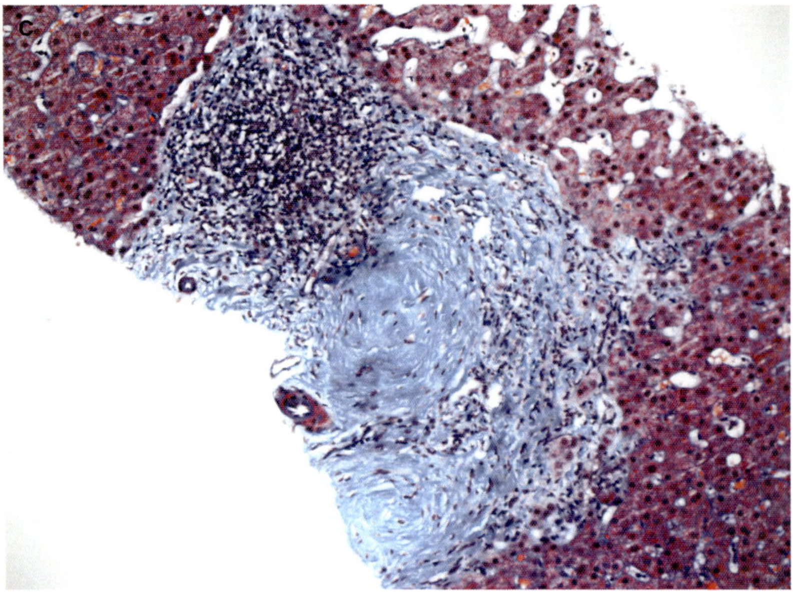

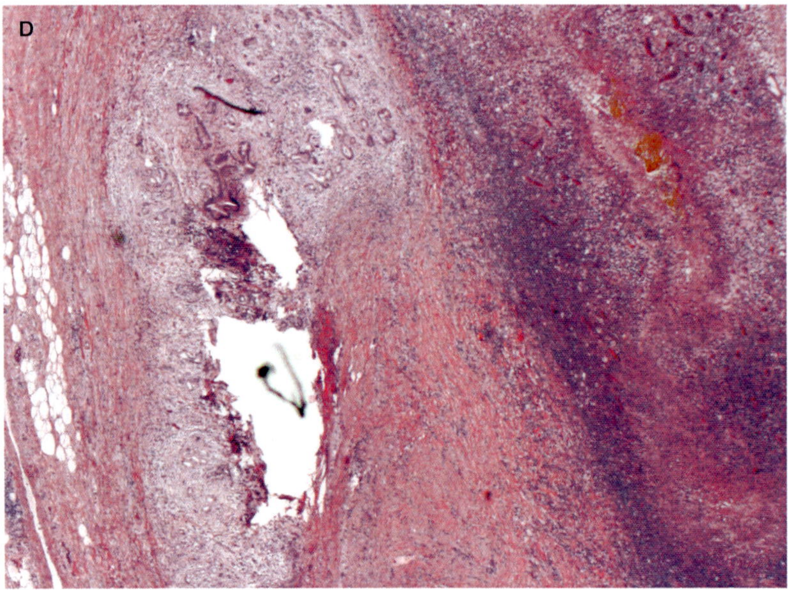

FIGURE 3-4

FIGURE 3-4 (C) Fibrous obliteration of bile duct (trichrome stain). (D) Extrahepatic bile duct showing ulceration and periductal abscess formation.

Overlap Syndrome

DEFINITION

Two immune-mediated liver diseases coexisting in the same patient either simultaneously or sequentially, including variants of AIH

CLINICAL FEATURES

- Predominantly AIH with secondary features that suggest an overlap with PBC, autoimmune cholangitis or PSC
- Diagnostic criteria for AIH + PBC

  AIH features (two out of three criteria required for the diagnosis):

  1. ALT levels greater than five times the upper limit of normal
  2. Serum IgG level greater than two times the upper limit of normal, or positive SMA
  3. Liver biopsy showing a chronic hepatitis pattern (Figure 3-5A)

  PBC features:

  1. Alkaline phosphatase levels greater than two times or gamma-glutamyl transpeptidase levels greater than five times the upper limit of normal
  2. Positive AMA
  3. Liver biopsy showing florid bile duct lesions (Figure 3-5B)

- AIH + PSC more commonly seen in pediatric patients

HISTOLOGIC FEATURE

- AIH + PBC: classic AIH and PBC-like bile duct injury; lobular hepatitis with acidophil bodies (not a feature of PBC but of AIH)
- AIH + PSC: classic AIH and varying degrees of bile duct injury. In pediatric patients the classic concentric fibrosis of PSC is rare. Any bile duct abnormality should raise the possibility for overlap syndrome in a pediatric patient with AIH

DIFFERENTIAL DIAGNOSIS

- Drug-induced liver injury
- Classic AIH
- PBC
- PSC

(continued)

Overlap Syndrome *(continued)*

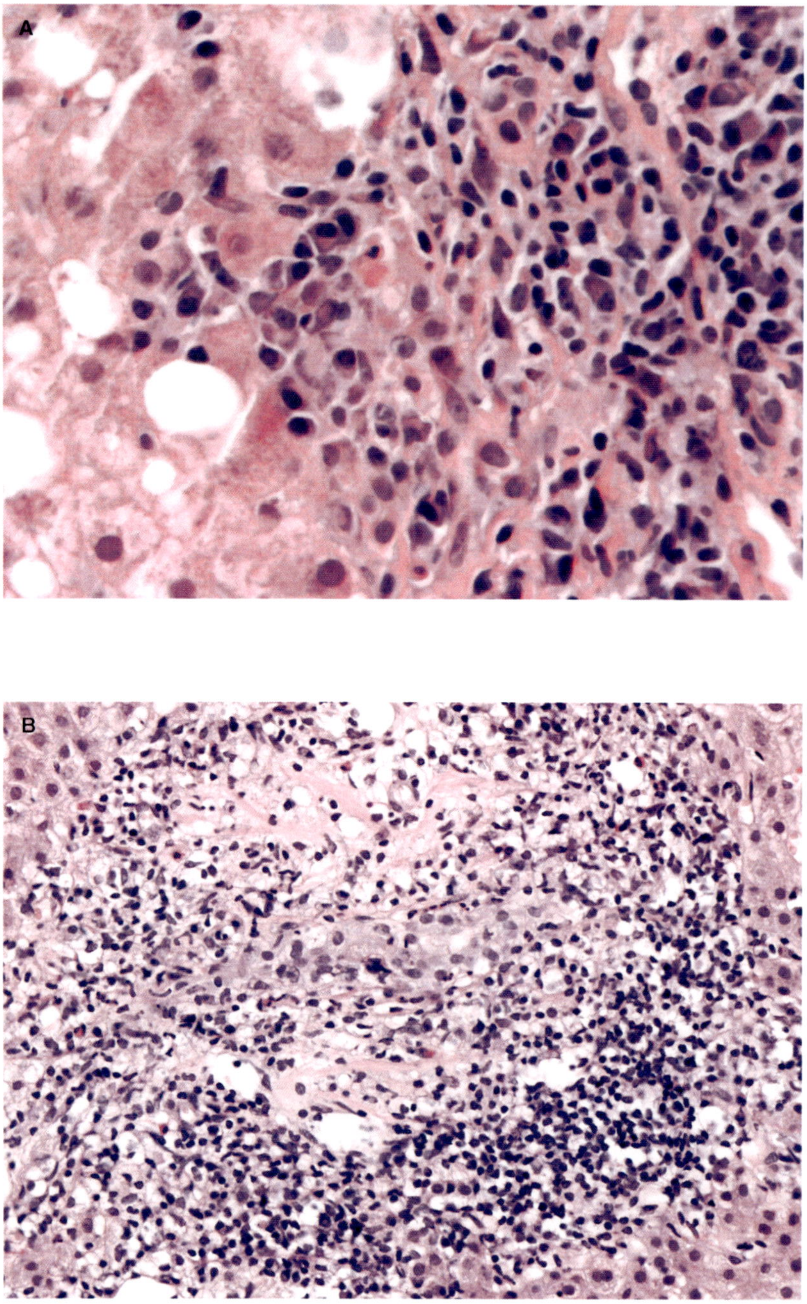

FIGURE 3-5

FIGURE 3-5 (A) Overlap syndrome. AIH with moderate lymphoplasmacytic infiltration. (B) Overlap syndrome. Florid bile duct lesion is present.

Metabolic and Hereditary Disorders

4

ALCOHOL-INDUCED LIVER DISEASE

NONALCOHOLIC STEATOHEPATITIS

HEREDITARY HEMOCHROMATOSIS

ALPHA-1-ANTITRYPSIN DEFICIENCY

Alcohol-Induced Liver Disease

DEFINITION

Hepatic injury due to chronic alcohol consumption

CLINICAL FEATURES

- Clinical manifestations range from asymptomatic disease to acute presentation with jaundice, fever, and hepatic decompensation
- Hepatomegaly

HISTOLOGIC FEATURES

- Steatosis (reversible with abstinence or "burnt-out"), macrovesicular, microvesicular or mixed, accentuated at the centrilobular zone (zone 3)
- Steatohepatitis, characterized by fatty change plus hepatocyte ballooning degeneration, Mallory-Denk bodies, lobular inflammation, and perivenular/pericellular fibrosis (Figures 4-1A, B)
- Alcoholic and nonalcoholic steatohepatitis (NASH) histologically indistinguishable in some cases
- Mallory-Denk body more prominent and more abundantly seen in alcoholic hepatitis
- Satellitosis, portal neutrophils, portal ductular proliferation, and cholestasis more frequently in alcoholic hepatitis than in NASH (Figure 4-1C)
- Mega-mitochondria: discrete round or oval intracytoplasmic inclusions in the perivenular hepatocytes (Figure 4-1D)
- Occasional extensive perivenular liver cell necrosis associated with deposition of fibrous tissue (sclerosing hyaline necrosis)
- Micronodular cirrhosis

DIFFERENTIAL DIAGNOSIS

- NASH
- Wilson's disease
- Drug-induced liver injury

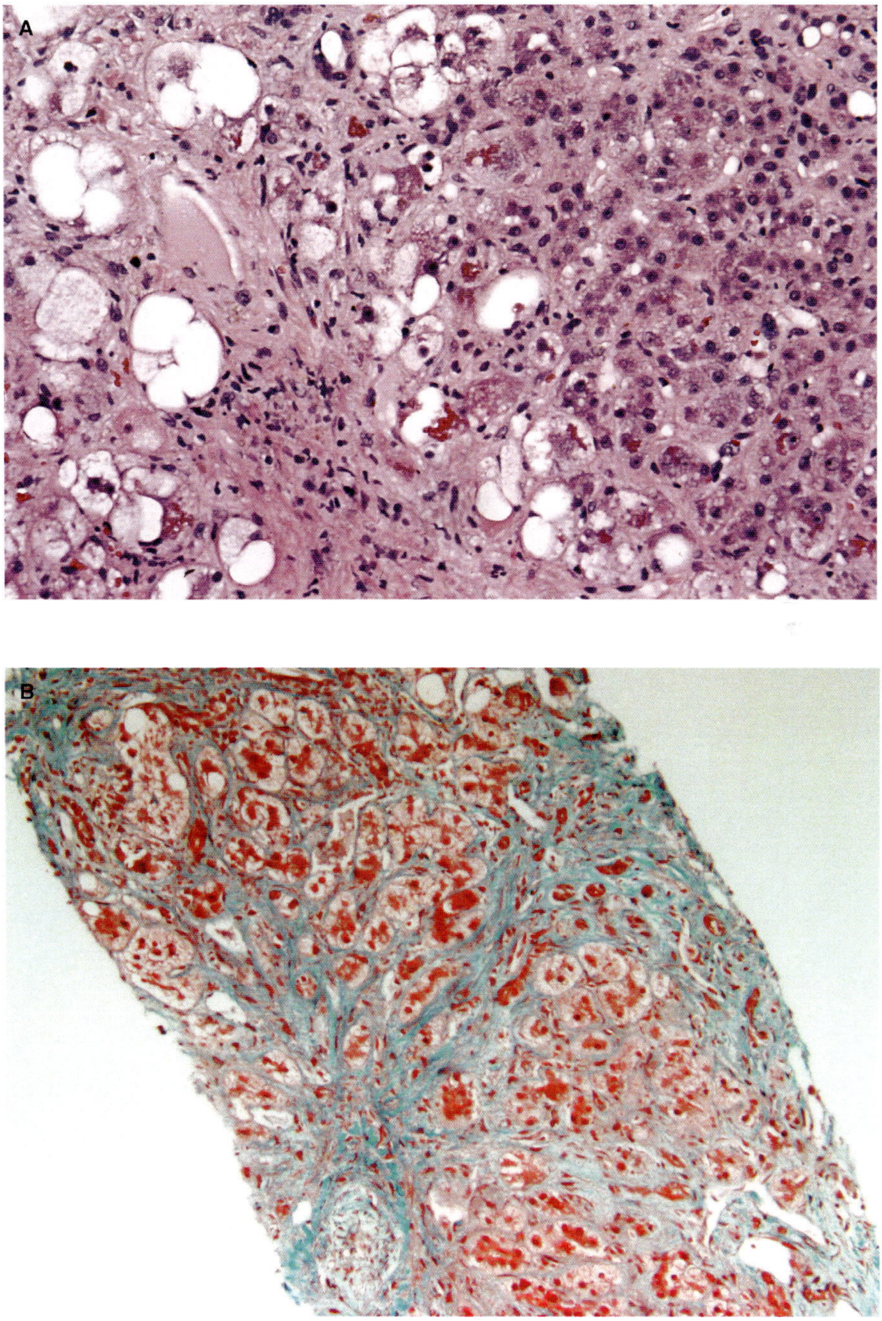

FIGURE 4-1

FIGURE 4-1 (A) Alcohol hepatitis. Hepatocytes contain numerous well-formed Mallory-Denk bodies. Lobular neutrophils are also noted. (B) Perivenular fibrosis. The central vein (lower left) is occlusive, and extensive sinusoidal fibrosis demonstrates an arachnoids pattern.

(*continued*)

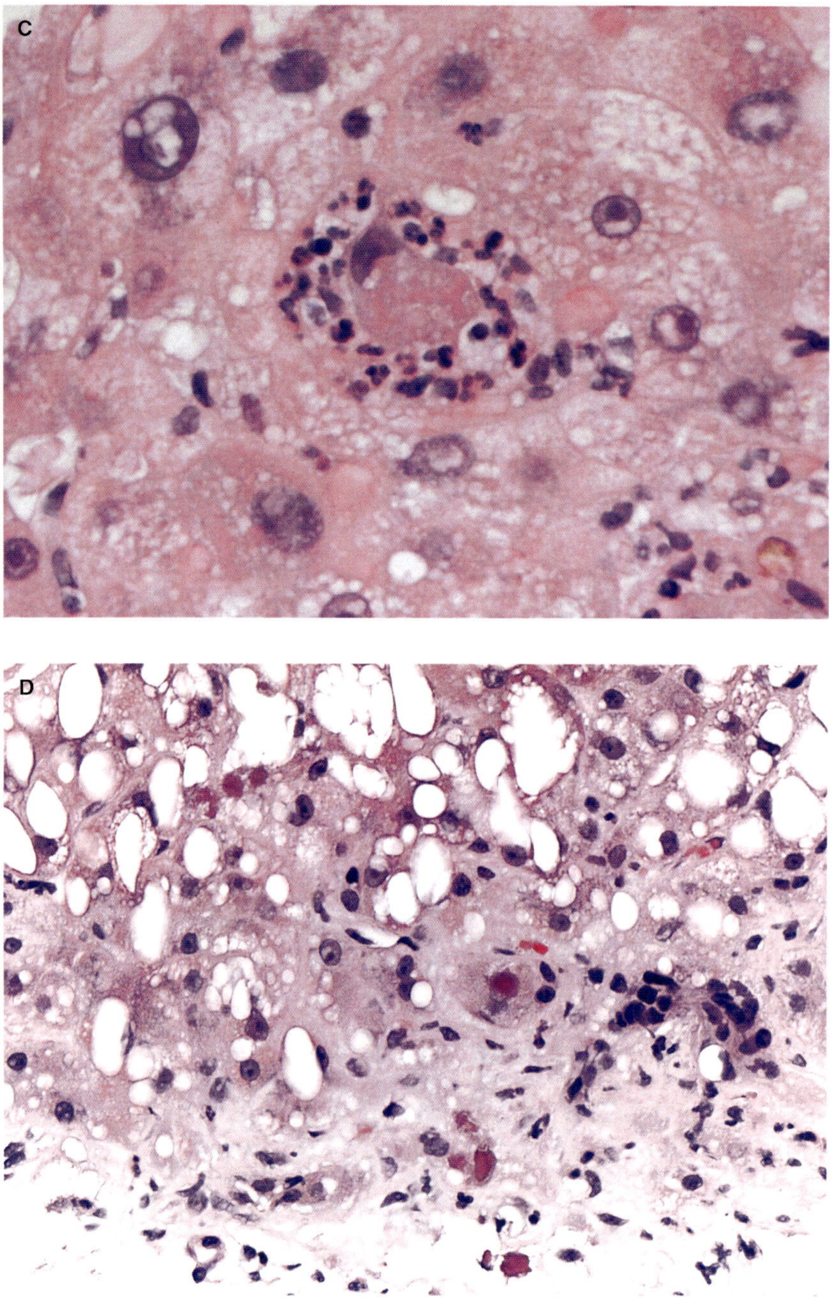

FIGURE 4-1

FIGURE 4-1 (C) Satellitosis: neutrophils surround a ballooned hepatocyte containing a Mallory-Denk body. This is more often seen in alcoholic steatohepatitis. (D) Megamitochondria: the same size or larger than the nucleus of hepatocytes, and distinctly round and eosinophilic.

Nonalcoholic Steatohepatitis

DEFINITION

Hepatic manifestation of metabolic syndrome of diabetes, obesity, hyperlipidemia, dyslipidemia, and malnutrition

CLINICAL FEATURES

- Usually asymptomatic
- Unexplained elevated liver enzymes and an abnormal imaging study are the most common reasons for coming to medical attention

HISTOLOGIC FEATURES

- Diagnosis mainly based on histology of liver biopsy
- Macrovesicular steatosis, ballooning degeneration, lobular inflammation with or without Mallory-Denk bodies and perivenular/pericellular fibrosis (Figures 4-2A, B, C, D)
- Lobular inflammation common and composed primarily of lymphocytes (prominent neutrophilic infiltrates more suggestive of alcoholic hepatitis)
- Glycogenated nuclei
- Commonly used grading and staging algorithms: Brunt system and the NASH clinical research network scoring system (CNR)
- Pediatric cases characterized by diffuse steatosis without zone 3 accentuation and more prominent portal inflammation and fibrosis; balloon degeneration and perisinusoidal fibrosis less typical

DIFFERENTIAL DIAGNOSIS

- Alcoholic liver disease
- Wilson's disease (pediatric patients)
- Drug-induced liver injury (amiodarone, steroids, L-asparaginase, tamoxifen, diltiazem, antiviral therapy for HIV, etc.)

(continued)

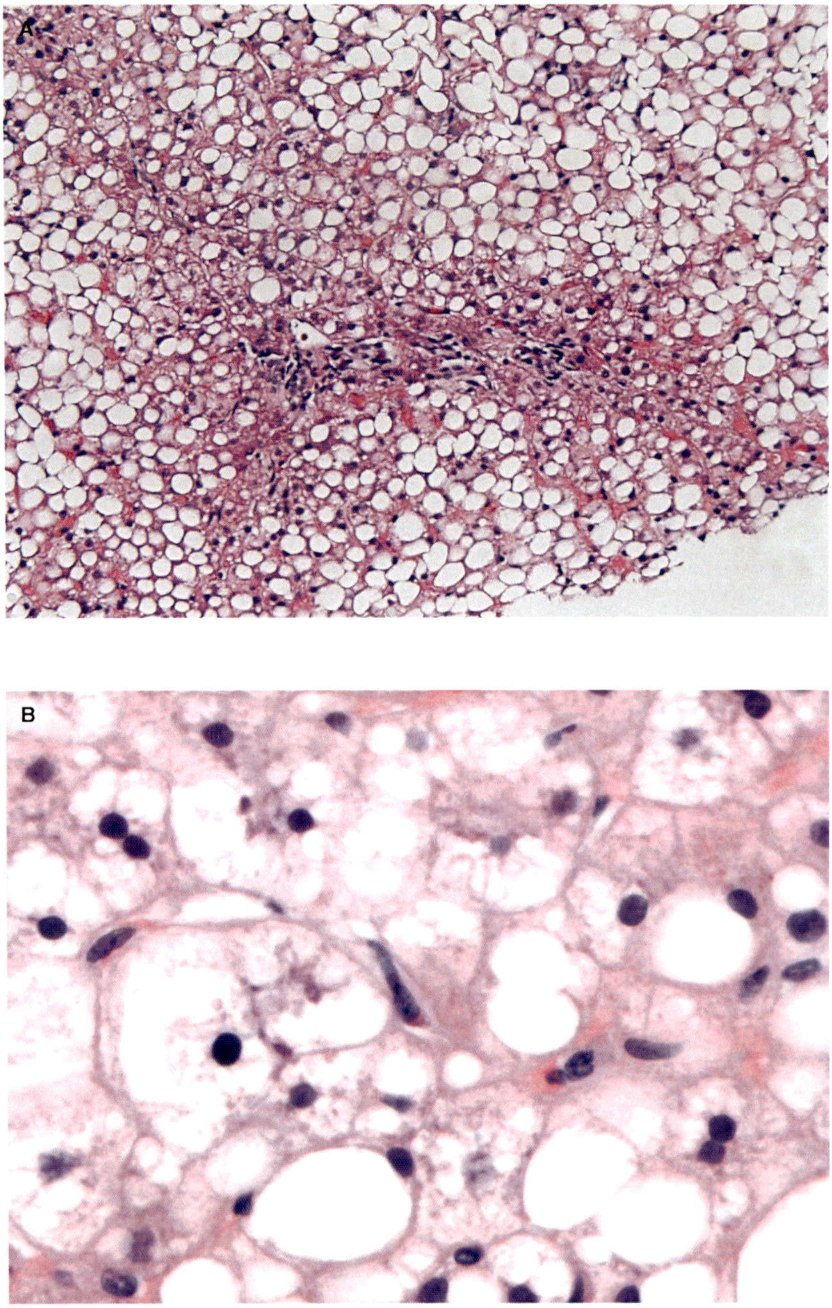

FIGURE 4-2

FIGURE 4-2 (A) Nonalcoholic fatty liver disease (NAFLD). Marked steatosis without ballooning degeneration. (B) Ballooned cells with ill-formed Mallory-Denk bodies.

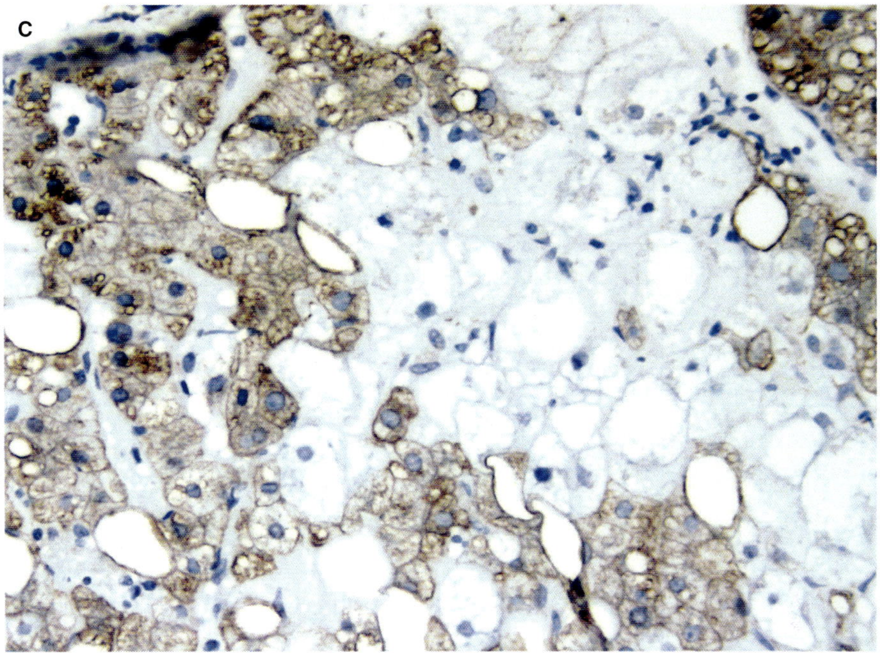

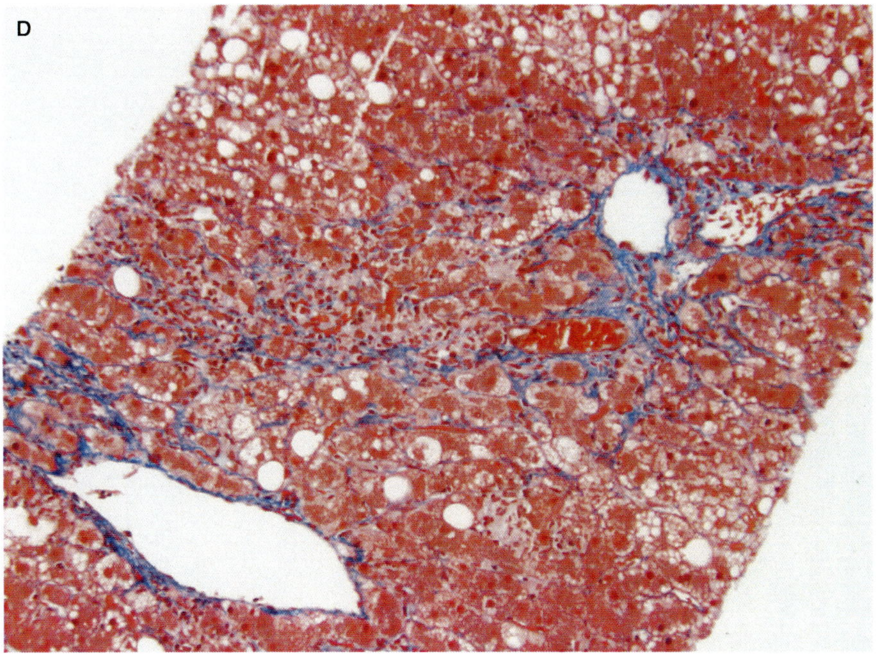

FIGURE 4-2

FIGURE 4-2 (C) Immunohistochemical stain for CK18 in NASH. Ballooning hepatocytes are negative for CK18 because of cytoskeletal damage. (D) Pericellular fibrosis in NASH. Fibrosis starts from the central vein and is present in a chicken-wire pattern.

Hereditary Hemochromatosis

DEFINITION

An autosomal recessive genetic disorder resulting in increased iron absorption from the gut, with deposition of iron in the parenchymal cells of the liver, heart, pancreas and other endocrine glands

CLINICAL FEATURES

- Most patients (85%) homozygous for C282Y mutation in the HFE gene (type 1)
- Most patients asymptomatic and identified by abnormal iron studies on routine screening chemistry panel or by screening family members of index patients
- Classic triad: cirrhosis, diabetes mellitus, skin pigmentation

HISTOLOGIC FINDINGS

- Iron accumulation initially in zone 1 hepatocytes, with clustering around bile canaliculi (Figures 4-3A, B)
- Iron accumulation in bile duct epithelium in advanced cases (Figure 4-3C)
- Quantitative iron performed on block useful in confirming the diagnosis
- Iron scoring system (Modified Scheuer's)

0. No visible iron
1. Some iron seen in zone 1 on high power
2. Iron granules easily seen in zone 1 on low power
3. Iron granules easily seen in zone 2
4. Iron granules seen with naked eye

DIFFERENTIAL DIAGNOSIS

- Secondary iron overload due to hemolysis, frequent blood transfusion, chronic liver disease (iron accumulation in Kupffer cells) (Figure 4-3D)

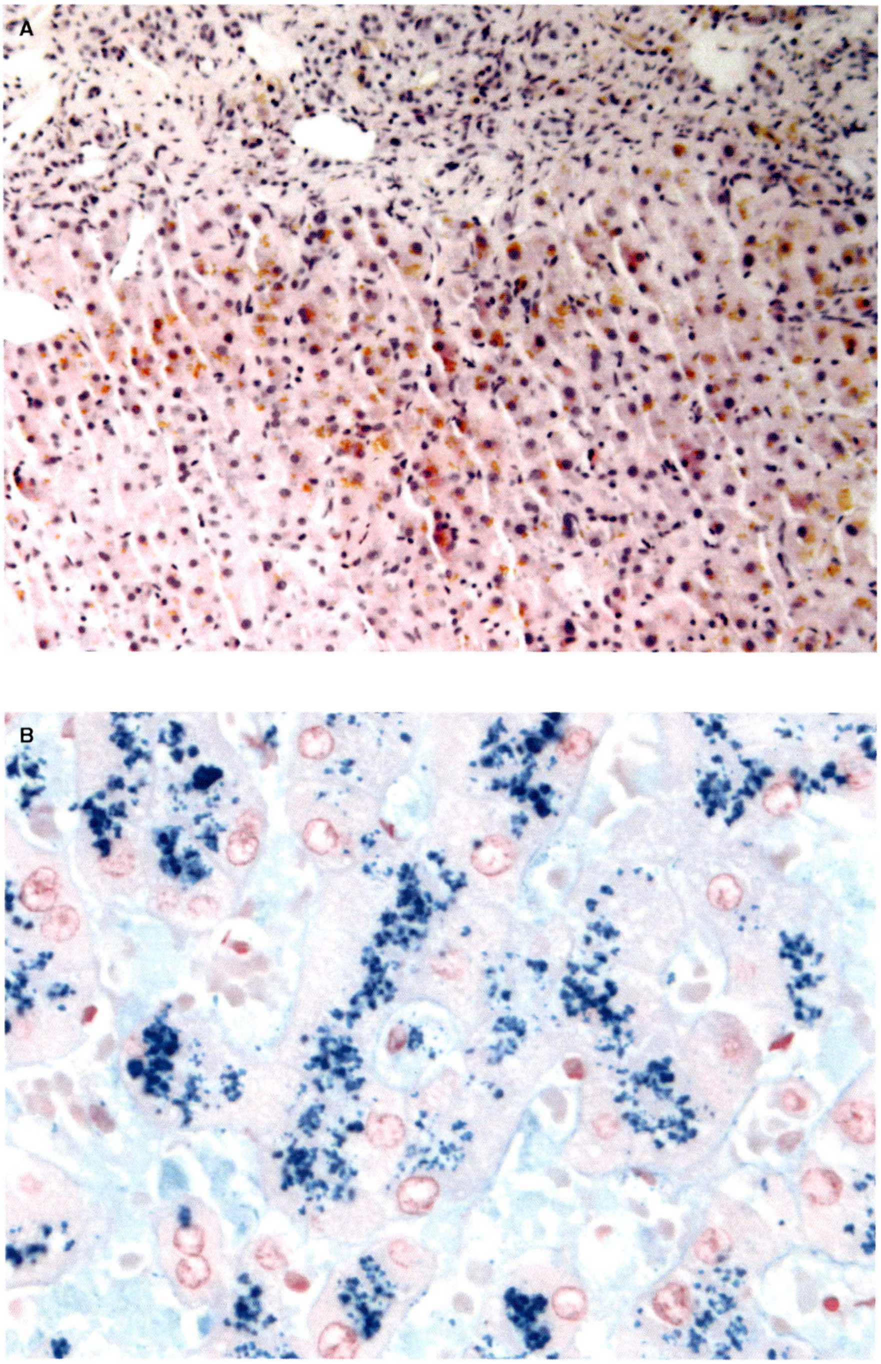

FIGURE 4-3

FIGURE 4-3 (A) Hemochromatosis (H&E). Golden pigment is accumulated in hepatocytes. (B) Perls' iron stain: iron accumulation in hepatocytes with a canalicular pattern.

(continued)

Hereditary Hemochromatosis *(continued)*

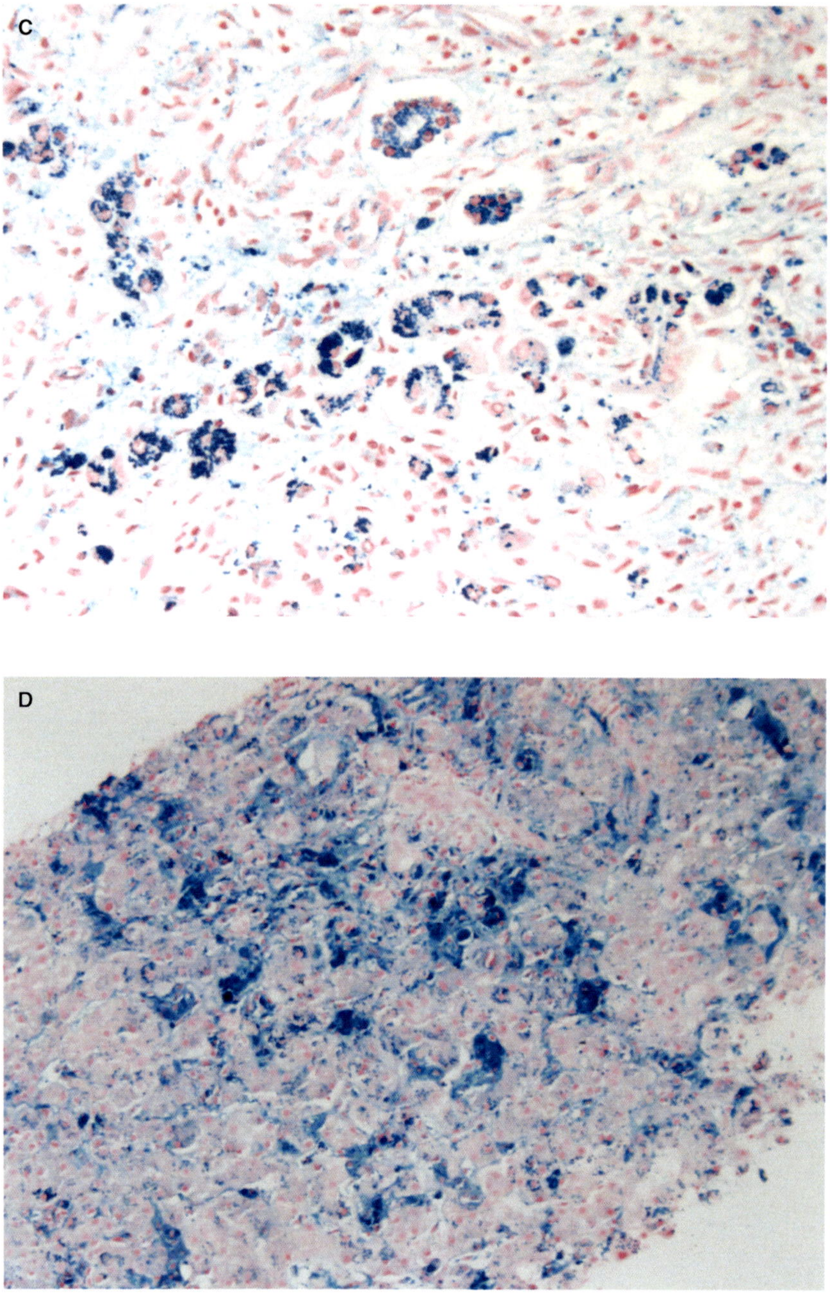

FIGURE 4-3

FIGURE 4-3 (C) Perls' iron stain: severe case with iron accumulation in biliary epithelium. (D) Hemosiderosis associated with sickle cell anemia (Perls' iron stain). Abundant hemosiderin in Kupffer cells and portal macrophages.

Alpha-1-Antitrypsin Deficiency

DEFINITION

Disorder associated with deficiency of alpha-1-antitrypsin (AAT), a serine proteinase inhibitor (Pi). The gene is located on chromosome 14q31-32; molecular abnormality leads to misfolding that prevents the transfer of protein from the rough to the smooth endoplasmic reticulum, and thus its release by hepatocytes.

CLINICAL FEATURES

- Panlobular emphysema and cirrhosis
- Bimodal distribution consists of neonatal hepatitis and chronic liver disease in adults
- Most common among people with northern European ancestry
- Normal gene product is PiM; most common deficiency alleles are PiS and PiZ
- PiZZ phenotype accounts for most severe cases
- Decreased serum AAT suggestive of the diagnosis; diagnosis confirmed by serum protein electrophoresis or DNA sequencing

PATHOLOGIC FEATURES

- PAS-positive, diastase-resistant globules in periportal hepatocytes (Figures 4-4A, B)
- Other than the globules, the histologic findings are nonspecific
- Globules difficult to detect in infants 12 weeks or younger
- Immunohistochemical staining for AAT may be helpful for ambiguous cases (Figure 4-4C)

DIFFERENTIAL DIAGNOSIS

- Neonatal hepatitis
- Extrahepatic biliary atresia
- TPN toxicity

(*continued*)

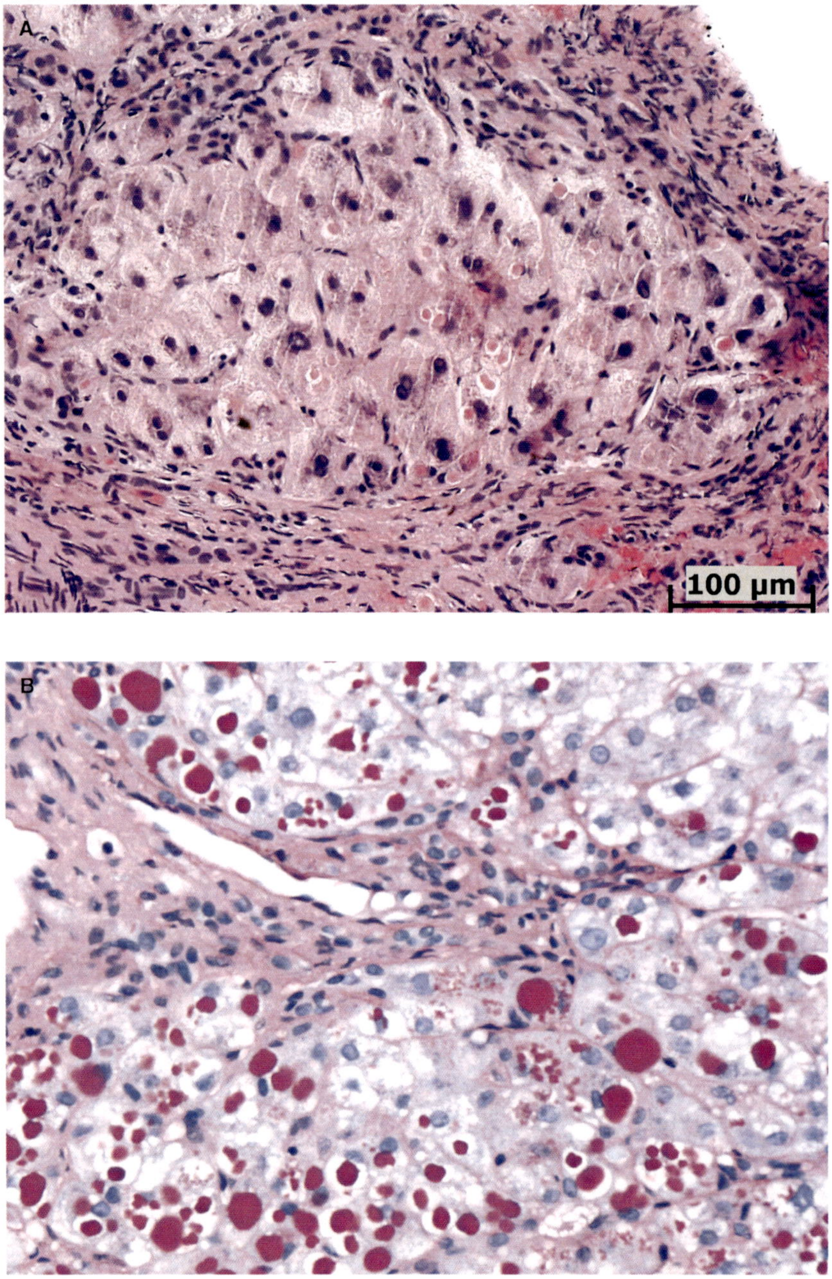

FIGURE 4-4

FIGURE 4-4 (A) AAT deficiency. Large hyaline globules are visible on H&E stained section in more advanced severe cases. (B) AAT globules. PAS-positive, diastase-resistant globules in periportal hepatocytes.

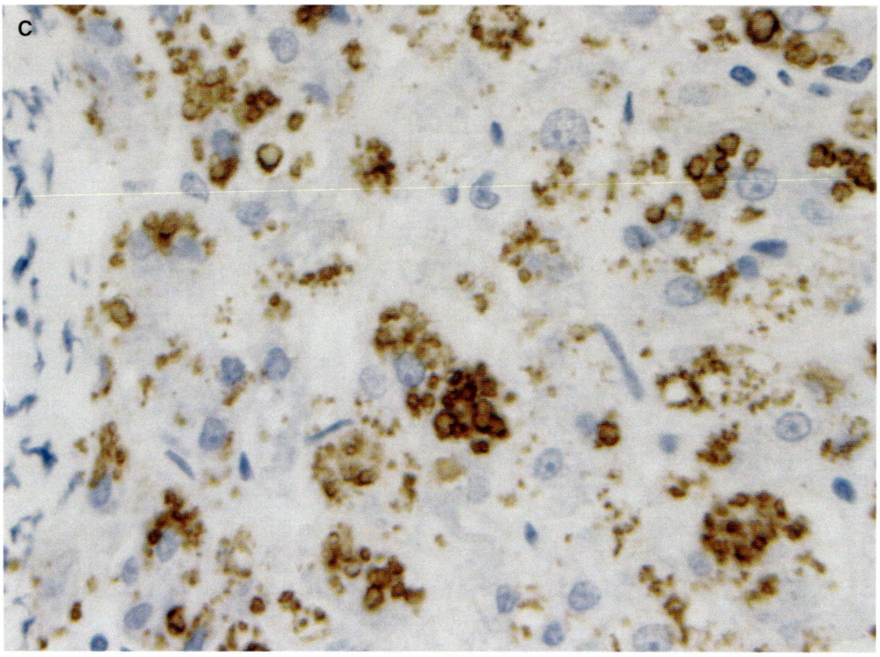

FIGURE 4-4

FIGURE 4-4 (C) Immunohistochemical stain for AAT.

5

Vascular Disorders

NONCIRRHOTIC PORTAL HYPERTENSION

BUDD-CHIARI SYNDROME (HEPATIC VEIN THROMBOSIS)

CARDIOGENIC HEPATIC CONGESTION

SINUSOIDAL OBSTRUCTION SYNDROME (VENO-OCCLUSIVE DISEASE)

AMYLOIDOSIS

Noncirrhotic Portal Hypertension

DEFINITION

Increase in portal pressure due to an intrahepatic or perihepatic lesion, in the absence of cirrhosis. Synonyms: noncirrhotic portal fibrosis, idiopathic portal hypertension, hepatoportal sclerosis

CLINICAL FEATURES

- Variable underlying etiology; possible causes include bacterial infection, toxin, and drugs, intrahepatic thrombosis or immunologic abnormalities
- More common in India and Japan
- Patients present with variceal bleeding and/or massive splenomegaly

PATHOLOGIC FEATURES

- Absence of cirrhosis
- Abnormal vascular architecture (approximation of or wide separation between central vein and portal tract) (Figure 5-1A)
- Portal vein obliteration with intimal thickening (Figure 5-1B)
- Aberrant vasculature such as dilated portal veins extending into lobule or herniation into hepatic parenchyma (Figure 5-1C)
- No evidence of hepatocellular injury

DIFFERENTIAL DIAGNOSIS

- Cirrhosis

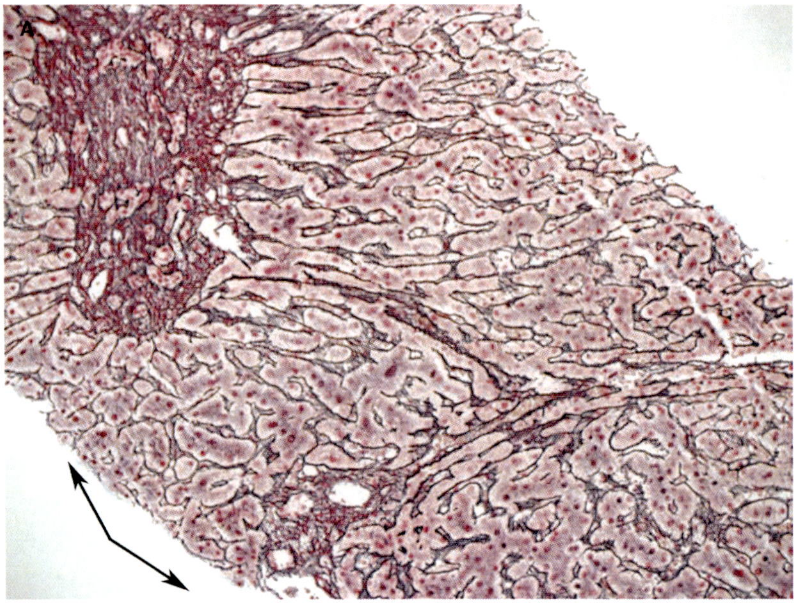

FIGURE 5-1

FIGURE 5-1 (A) Reticulin stain highlights the abnormal approximation of portal tracts (arrow), and focal nodular pattern (lower right aspect).

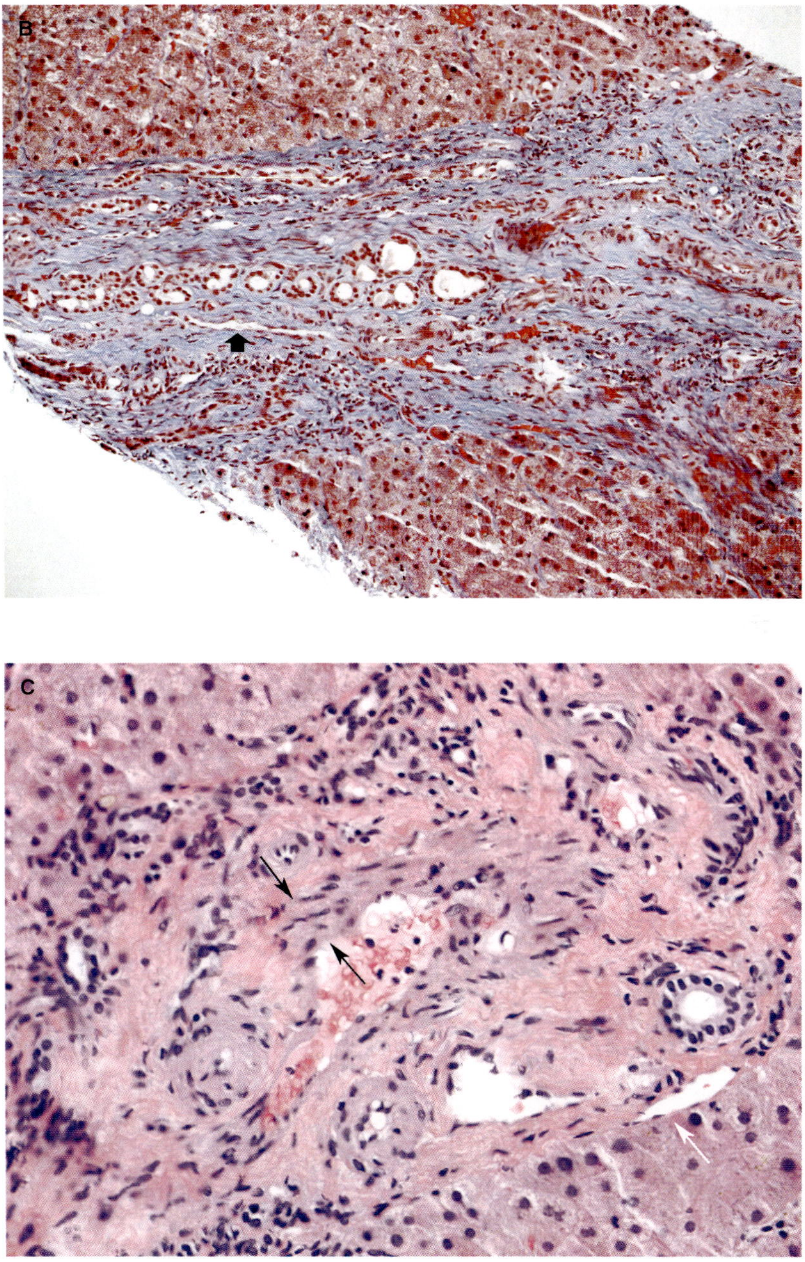

FIGURE 5-1

FIGURE 5-1 (B) A portal area with fibrotic expansion in a noncirrhotic liver. The portal vein is narrow and obliterated (arrow). (C) Intimal thickening in a portal vein (black arrows). Hepatic arterioles are unremarkable. A dilated portal vein extending into the lobules is also present (white arrow).

Budd-Chiari Syndrome (Hepatic Vein Thrombosis)

DEFINITION

A heterogeneous group of disorders characterized by hepatic venous outflow obstruction. Classic Budd-Chiari syndrome results from thrombosis of one or more hepatic veins at their openings into the inferior vena cava. However, obstruction can occur anywhere from the right atrium to the small hepatic venules.

CLINICAL FEATURES

- Etiologies include hypercoagulable status, infections, malignancies, and miscellaneous conditions
- Abdominal pain, tender hepatomegaly, ascites
- Diagnosis made by venography or less invasive radiologic imaging including Doppler ultrasonography, magnetic resonance imaging, and computed tomography

PATHOLOGIC FEATURES

- Sinusoidal dilatation, congestion, and hemorrhage (acute phase) (Figures 5-2A, B)
- Red-cell trabecular lesion (red blood cell extravasation, or red blood cells replacing damaged hepatocytes that have undergone anoxic ischemic necrosis) (Figure 5-2C)
- Sinusoidal fibrosis (chronic phase) (Figure 5-2D)

DIFFERENTIAL DIAGNOSIS

- Venous congestion secondary to congestive heart failure
- Sinusoidal obstruction syndrome

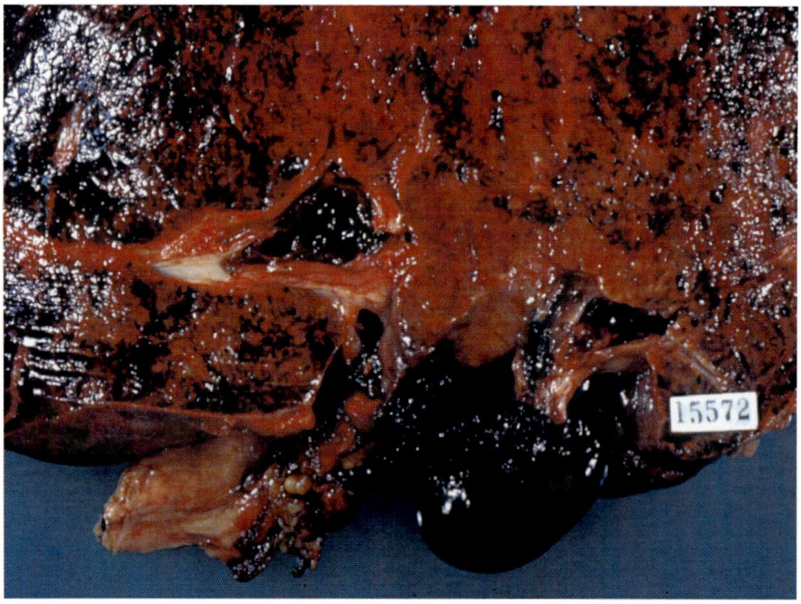

FIGURE 5-2

FIGURE 5-2 (A) Budd-Chiari syndrome due to thrombsis of a large hepatic vein. The background parenchyma is congested and hemorrhagic.

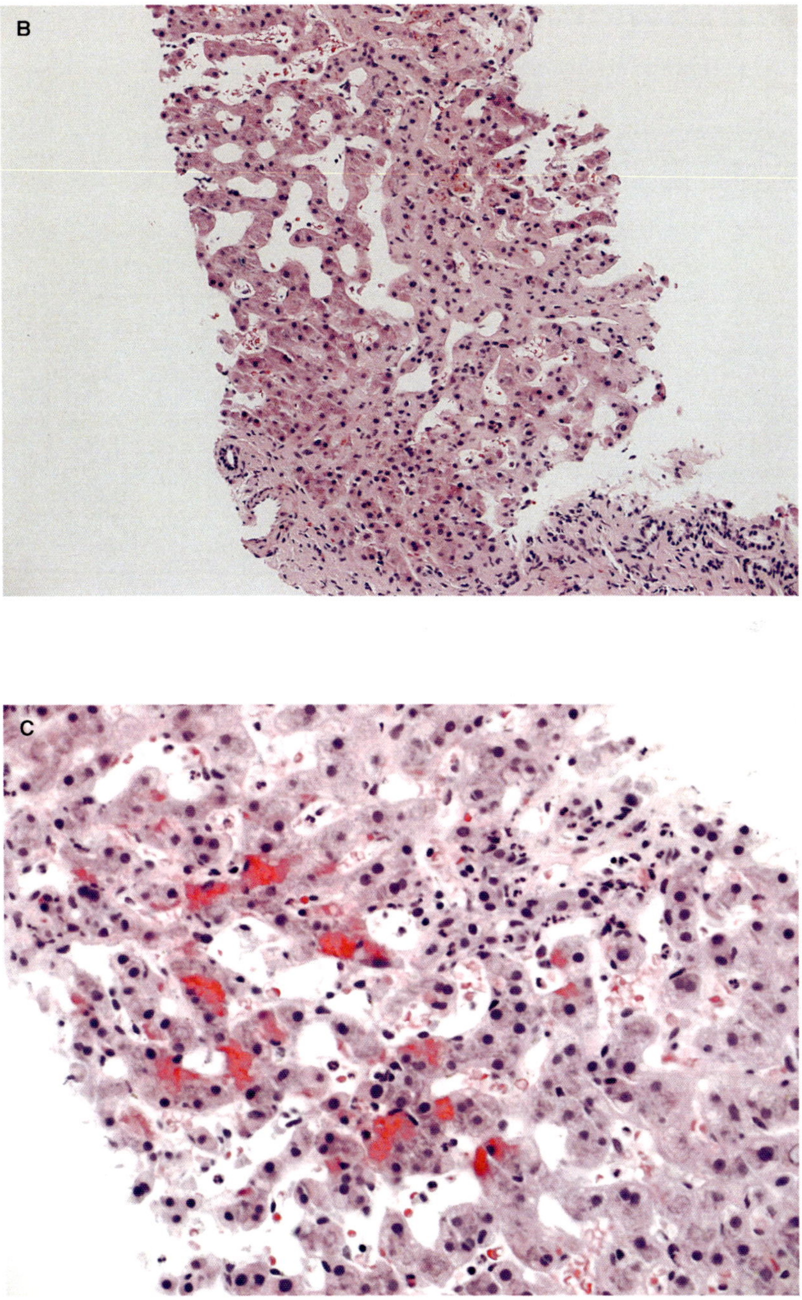

FIGURE 5-2

FIGURE 5-2 (B) Sinusoidal dilatation in zone 3 with red cell extravasation. (C) Hepatic cords show atrophy, and red cells replace damaged hepatocytes (red-cell trabecular lesion).

(continued)

Budd-Chiari Syndrome (Hepatic Vein Thrombosis) *(continued)*

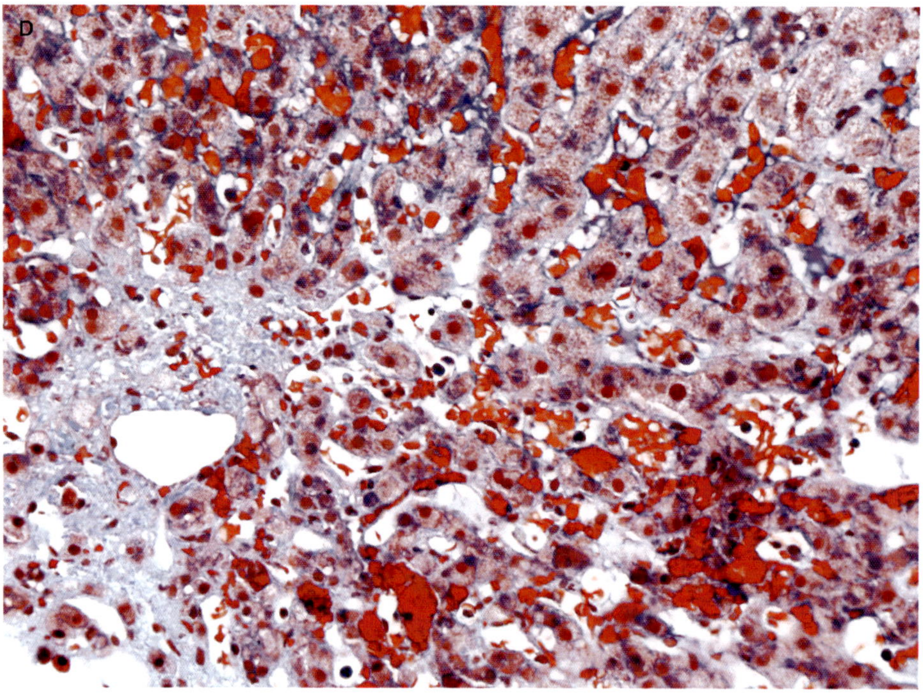

FIGURE 5-2

FIGURE 5-2 (D) Trichrome stain highlights sinusoidal fibrosis. Hepatocyte necrosis is noted around central vein.

Cardiogenic Hepatic Congestion

DEFINITION

Passive hepatic congestion due to reduced cardiac function or heart failure; the latter leads to increased hepatic venous pressure, decreased blood outflow, and decreased intrahepatic oxygen saturation.

CLINICAL FEATURES

- Etiologies include cardiomyopathy with heart failure, tricuspid valve disease, constrictive pericarditis and so on
- Symptoms: hepatomegaly with dull right upper quadrant pain

HISTOLOGIC FEATURES

- Sinusoidal dilatation and centrilobular fibrosis
- Atrophy of hepatocytes in zone 3 extending to zone 2 (Figure 5-3A)
- Cardiac cirrhosis (Figure 5-3B)

DIFFERENTIAL DIAGNOSIS

- Budd-Chiari syndrome (hepatic vein thrombosis)
- Sinusoidal obstruction syndrome

(*continued*)

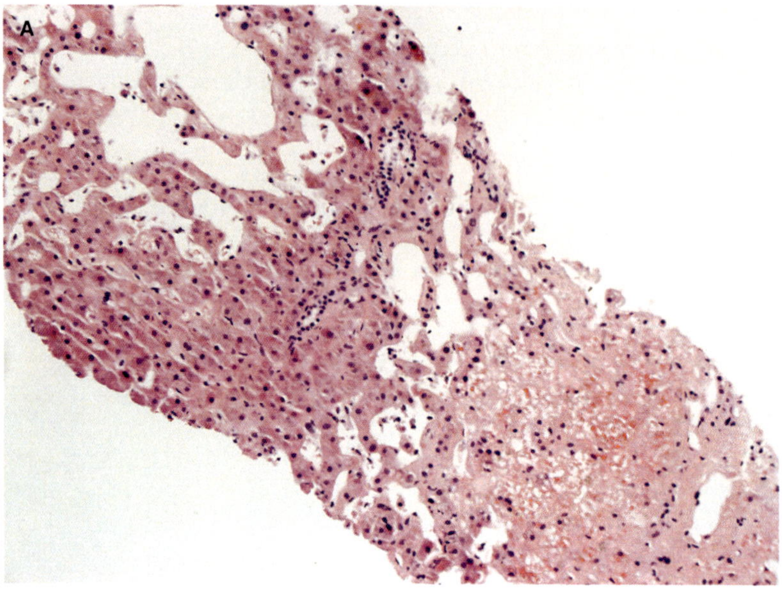

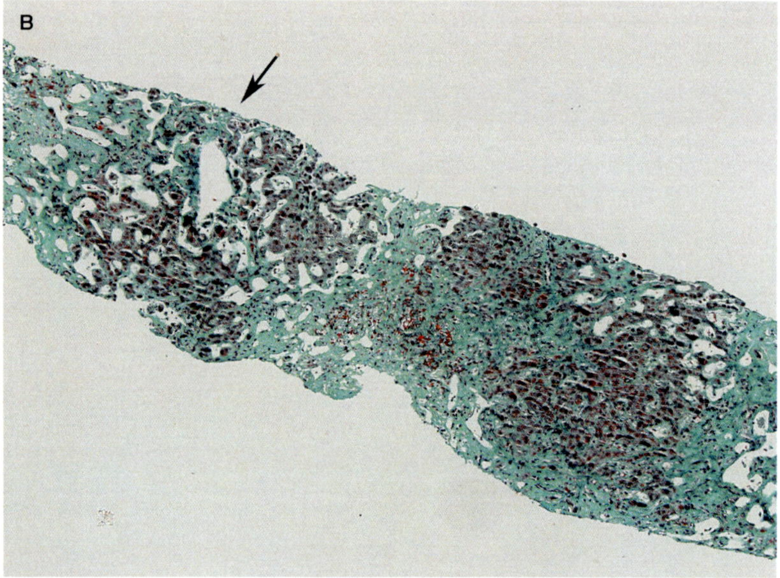

FIGURE 5-3

FIGURE 5-3 (A) Sinusoidal dilatation, congestion and hepatocyte dropout in the centrilobular area. Hepatocytes around the portal triads are preserved. (B) Cardiac cirrhosis. Uninvolved portal vein (arrow) is centrally located in the nodule (reverse lobulation).

Sinusoidal Obstruction Syndrome (Veno-Occlusive Disease)

DEFINITION

A form of toxic liver injury characterized histologically by diffuse damage of centrilobular hepatocytes. The primary site of the toxic injury is likely the sinusoidal endothelial cells. Sinusoidal obstruction syndrome (SOS) is currently the preferred term.

CLINICAL FEATURES

- Most common cause is stem cell transplantation and high-dose chemotherapy, but other etiologies include chemotherapy, radiation, and herbal medicine; originally described in Jamaican drinkers of pyrrolizidine alkaloid-containing bush tea
- Symptoms: tender hepatomegaly, fluid retention and weight gain and elevated serum bilirubin that follow cytoreductive chemotherapy

HISTOLOGIC FEATURES

- First recognizable histologic change is widening of the subendothelial zone
- Dilation and engorgement of sinusoids, extravasation of red cells through the space of Disse, and frank necrosis of perivenular hepatocytes (Figure 5-4A)
- Fibrotic obliteration of terminal hepatic veins may be seen (Figures 5-4B, C)

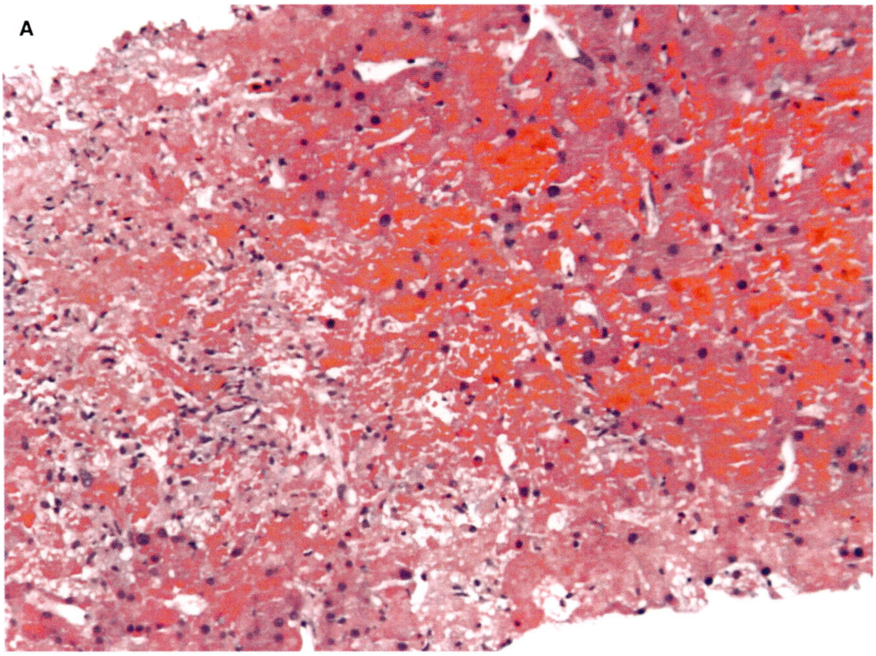

FIGURE 5-4

FIGURE 5-4 (A) Veno-occlusive disease. Marked congestion, hemorrhage, and hepatic cord atrophy.

(continued)

Sinusoidal Obstruction Syndrome (Veno-Occlusive Disease) *(continued)*

DIFFERENTIAL DIAGNOSIS

- Hepatic congestion secondary to cardiac failure
- Budd-Chiari syndrome (hepatic vein thrombosis)
- Acute graft versus host disease

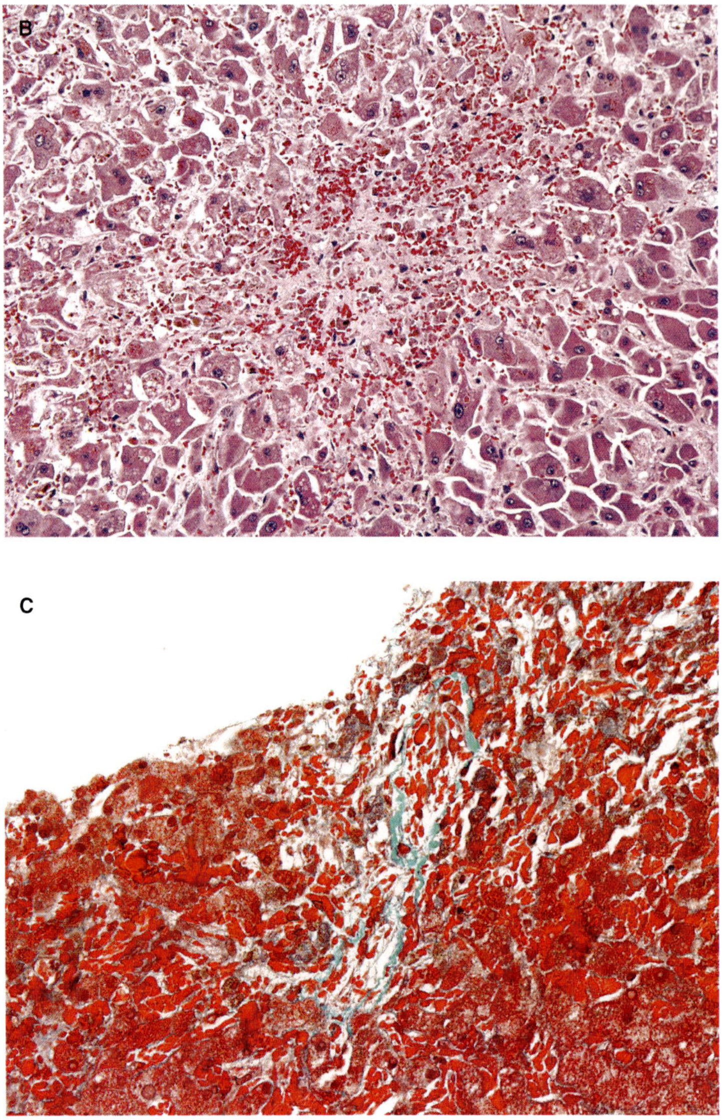

FIGURE 5-4

FIGURE 5-4 (B) Terminal hepatic venule (central vein) with fibrous obliterans. (C) Trichrome stain highlights an occluded central vein. Marked congestion is noted in the sinusoids.

Amyloidosis

DEFINITION
Extracellular deposition of amyloid consisting of fibril protein (95%), glycoproteins, and P comportment. Amyloidosis is divided into (1) primary amyloidosis (AL) (immunoglobulin light chain) associated, (2) secondary amyloidosis SAA (serum amyloid protein) related, (3) localized tumor-forming amyloidosis, and (4) familial amyloidosis.

CLINICAL FEATURES
- Fatigue, weight loss and edema, jaundice, hepatomegaly
- Significant hemorrhage may occcur following liver biopsy
- portal hypertension rare

HISTOLOGIC FEATURES
- Deposition of homogeneous amorphous material in the sinusoids, space of Disse and vascular wall (Figure 5-5A)
- Congo red stain demonstrating orange-colored staining with green birefringence with polarized light (Figure 5-5B)

DIFFERENTIAL DIAGNOSIS
- Monoclonal protein (M-protein) as tissue deposition

(*continued*)

Amyloidosis *(continued)*

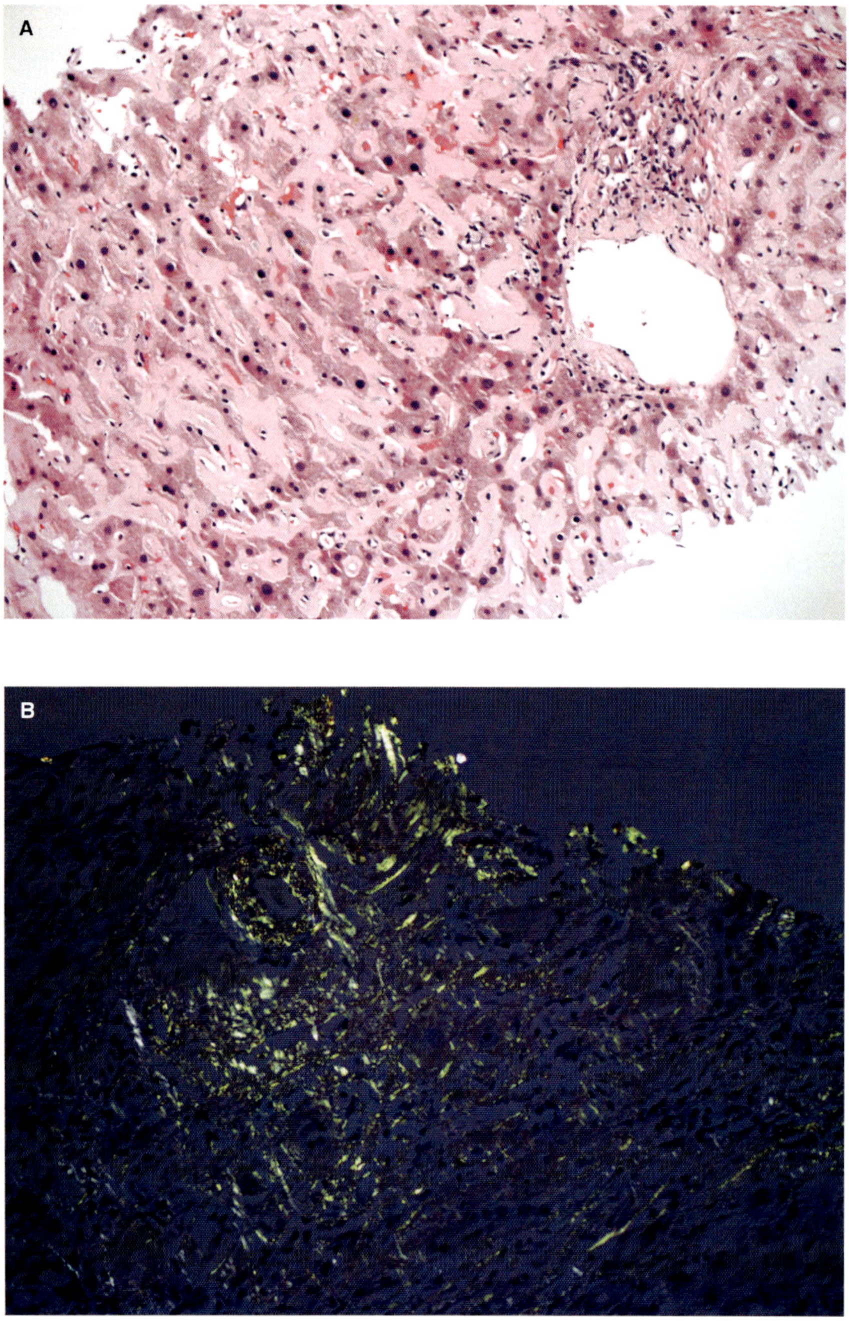

FIGURE 5-5

FIGURE 5-5 (A) Deposition of homogeneous amorphous material is present in the sinusoidal area. (B) Congo red stain shows apple-green birefringence in congophilic area.

6

Neonatal Disorders

NEONATAL HEPATITIS

PAUCITY OF INTRAHEPATIC BILE DUCTS

EXTRAHEPATIC BILIARY ATRESIA (EBA)

Neonatal Hepatitis

DEFINITION

A neonatal liver disease characterized by cholestasis and inflammation. About 40% of cases are idiopathic; other cases may be caused by infectious or metabolic disorders. A generic term *neonatal hepatitis syndrome* (NHS) has been used to refer to these conditions.

CLINICAL FEATURES

- Neonatal cholestasis, mainly of conjugated bilirubin
- Congenital infections seen in some cases: cytomegalovirus (CMV), rubella virus, herpes simplex virus (HSV), varicella-zoster virus (VZV), Coxsackie virus, *Treponema pallidum*, or *Toxoplasmosis*
- Initially, may be extremely challenging to distinguish from other neonatal cholestatic conditions discussed in this chapter

PATHOLOGIC FINDINGS

- Hepatomegaly common
- Microscopically, portal tracts exhibit a mixed inflammatory cellular infiltration, and lobular inflammation present to a lesser extent (Figure 6-1A)
- Degenerative changes of hepatocytes including swelling and ballooning, prominent giant cell transformation (multinucleated hepatocytes) (Figure 6-1B)
- Cholestasis
- Paucity of interlobular bile ducts can also be seen
- Fibrosis may occur in some cases

DIFFERENTIAL DIAGNOSIS

- Biliary atresia (BA)
- Alpha-1-antitrypsin deficiency
- Paucity of intrahepatic bile ducts (PIBD)
- Type 1 tyrosinemia
- Genetic syndromes of cholestasis and other metabolic diseases

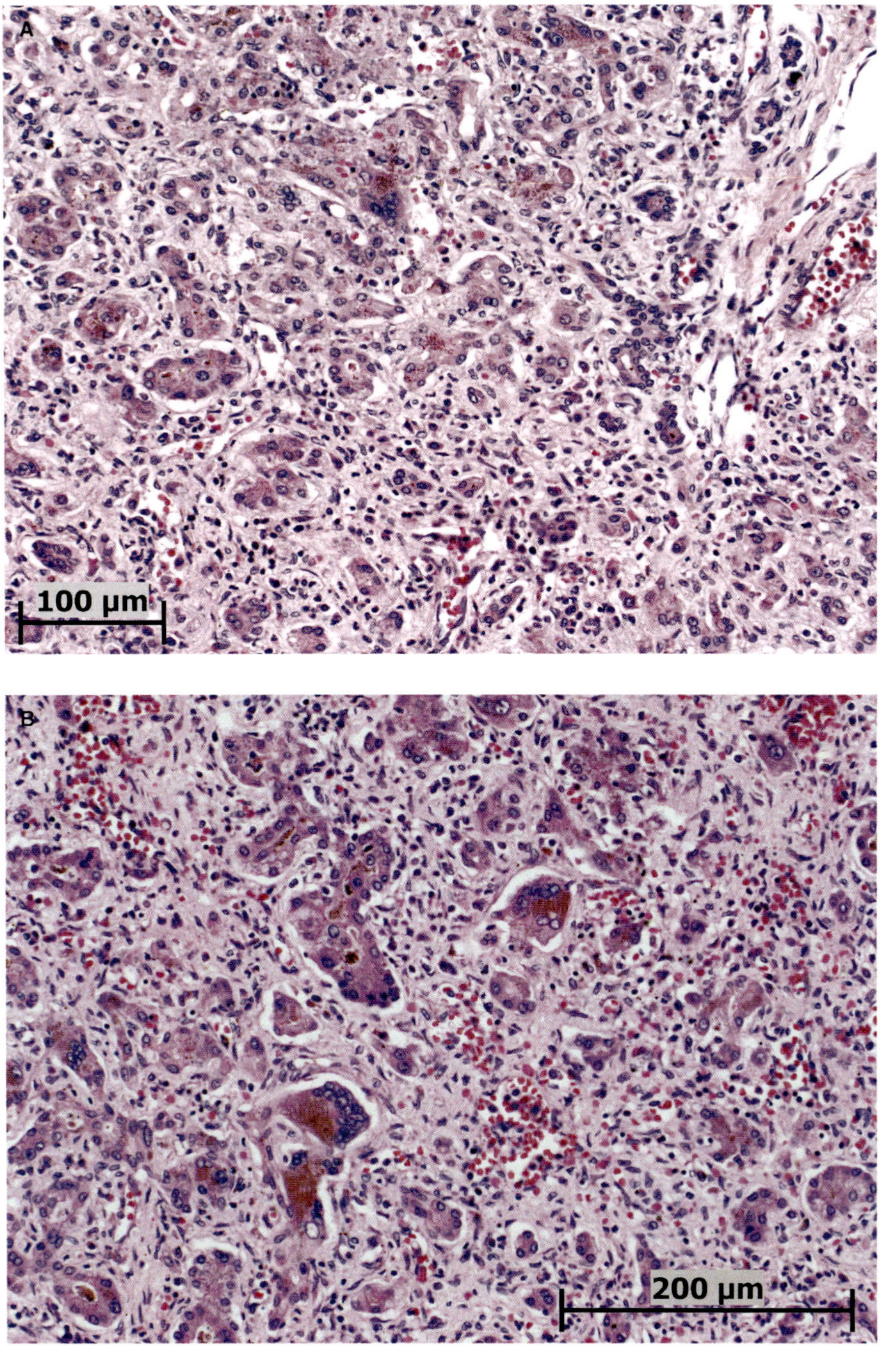

FIGURE 6-1

FIGURE 6-1 (A) Neonatal hepatitis (NH). There are portal and lobular inflammatory cellular infiltrates, extensive pericellular fibrosis, and canalicular cholestasis. There is focal hepatocytic rosette formation. Extramedullary hematopoiesis is evident.
(B) Multinucleated giant hepatocytes are frequently seen, thus the name "giant cell hepatitis."

Paucity of Intrahepatic Bile Ducts

DEFINITION

A group of disorders with the common pathologic denominator of *reduced number of intrahepatic bile ducts*. In the context of this chapter, PIBD refers to two categories of disorders: Alagille syndrome (AGS) and nonsyndromic PIBD in infants and children. AGS, *aka* arteriohepatic dysplasia, is a congenital malformation involving multiple systems. The etiology of nonsyndromic PIBD is largely unknown but some cases may be associated with congenital infection (e.g., CMV, rubella virus), alpha-1-antitrypsin deficiency, or other inborn errors of bile acid metabolism.

CLINICAL FEATURES

ALAGILLE SYNDROME

- Underlying genetic abnormality: mutations of *JAG1* (a gene coding ligand for the NOTCH1 receptor), which may be autosomal dominant (AD)-inherited; around 60% of patients have de novo mutations
- Combination of cholestasis, pulmonary artery stenosis, and special facial features of inverted triangle-shaped, deep-set eyes, prominent forehead, and pointed nose
- Endoscopic retrograde cholangiopancreatography (ERCP) may reveal narrowing of extrahepatic biliary tree (due to bile duct hypoplasia in some patients) or intrahepatic bile ducts

NONSYNDROMIC PAUCITY OF INTRAHEPATIC BILE DUCTS

- No associated extrahepatic disease
- Clinical outcome worse, with many patients presenting with progressive cholestasis and severe pruritus

PATHOLOGIC FEATURES

- A spectrum of changes, including mild portal inflammation and lack of normal appearing centrally located open bile ducts (Figures 6-2A and B).
- At 3 to 6 months of age, there may be ongoing bile duct injury and giant-cell transformation.
- Loss of bile duct starts in early infancy and progresses into childhood.
- Careful assessment of well-oriented portal tracts is required for diagnosis, in order to record number of open or normal interlobular bile ducts. The average number of interlobular bile ducts per portal tract cross section is 0.9 to 1.8. If more than five portal tracts can be evaluated in a biopsy and the ratio is less than 0.5, PIBD can be diagnosed.

DIFFERENTIAL DIAGNOSIS

- Pitfall: BD/portal tract ratio of 0.5 may be seen in premature babies with cholestasis as part of a physiologic cholestasis, and should not be interpreted as PIBD.
- Other diseases may cause paucity of bile ducts in later stages, such as extrahepatic BA, Langerhans histiocytosis, sclerosing cholangitis, and primary biliary cirrhosis. The latter two are usually not a concern in the differential as they develop later in life.

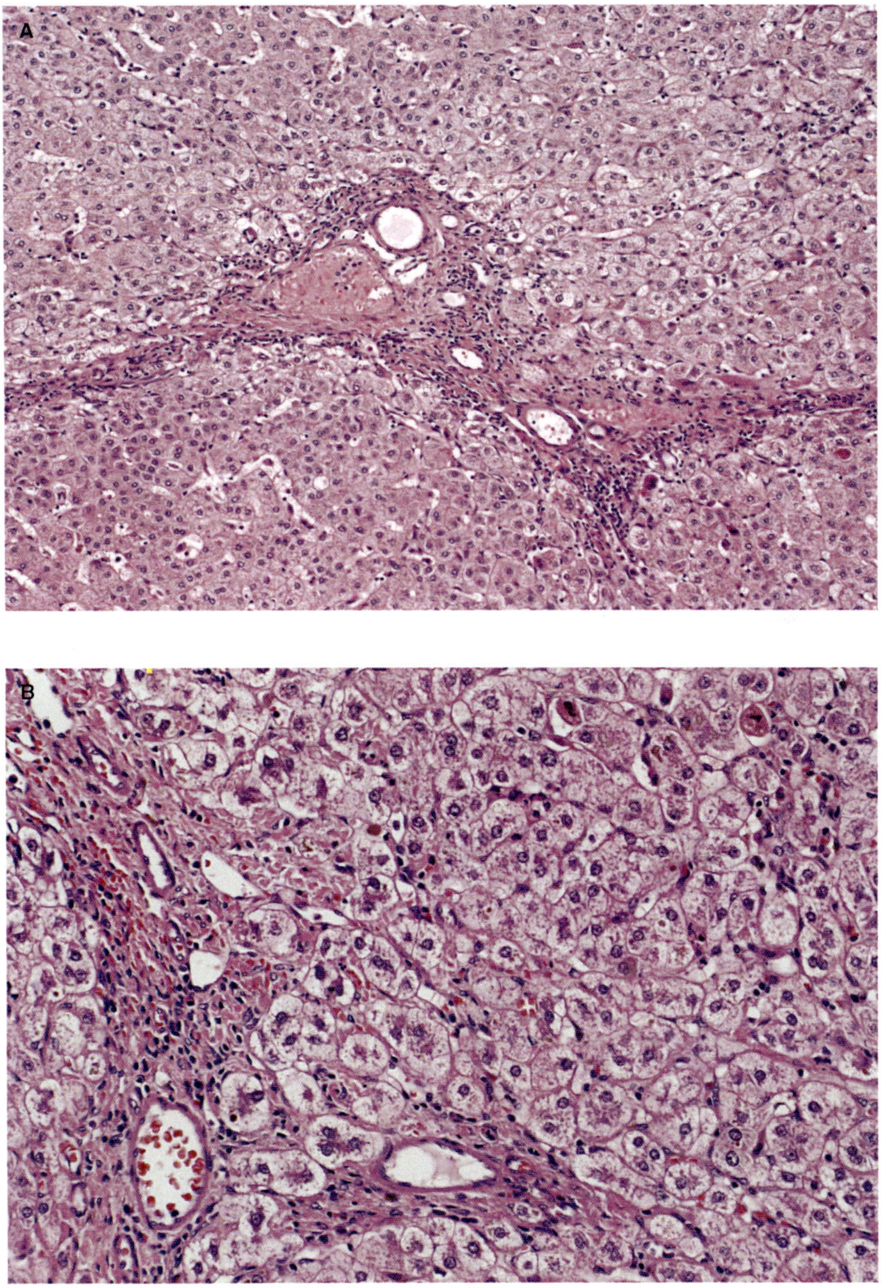

FIGURE 6-2

FIGURE 6-2 (A) AGS. The portal tracts contain no bile ducts. There is minimal lymphocytic infiltration. The background liver architecture is otherwise unremarkable. (B) Same case as Figure 6-2A. High magnification shows portal tract containing several hepatic arteries but no accompanying bile duct. There is mild fibrosis and minimal lymphocytic infiltration. The liver parenchyma contains occasional acidophil bodies.

Extrahepatic Biliary Atresia (EBA)

DEFINITION

Total or segmental atresia of the extrahepatic bile ducts of unknown etiology. The main significance of making the diagnosis early is the potential benefit from the *Kasai* procedure (hepatic portoenterostomy), a palliative surgery, which delays the progression of liver disease. Good long-term prognosis may be achieved if the procedure is done within the first 2 months of life. However, since the underlying pathogenesis will continue to progressively damage the intrahepatic bile ducts, leading to biliary cirrhosis, liver transplantation is the only curative treatment.

CLINICAL FEATURES

- Persistent neonatal cholestasis

PATHOLOGIC FEATURES

- End-stage disease characterized by extensive fibrosis or cirrhosis (Figure 6-3A)
- Various segments of the biliary tree may be involved (Figure 6-3B), with lack or attenuation of ductal epithelium (Figure 6-3C)
- Portal tract inflammation and/or edema, ductular proliferation, dilated bile ducts (Figure 6-3D)
- Hepatocytic and canalicular cholestasis (often with bile plugs)
- May have giant cell transformation and extramedullary hematopoiesis
- PIBD developing gradually with disease progression
- Diagnosis requires close correlation with clinical history and imaging studies, including ERCP

DIFFERENTIAL DIAGNOSIS

- Other diseases causing biliary obstruction: choledochal cyst
- NH
- Syndromic PIBD

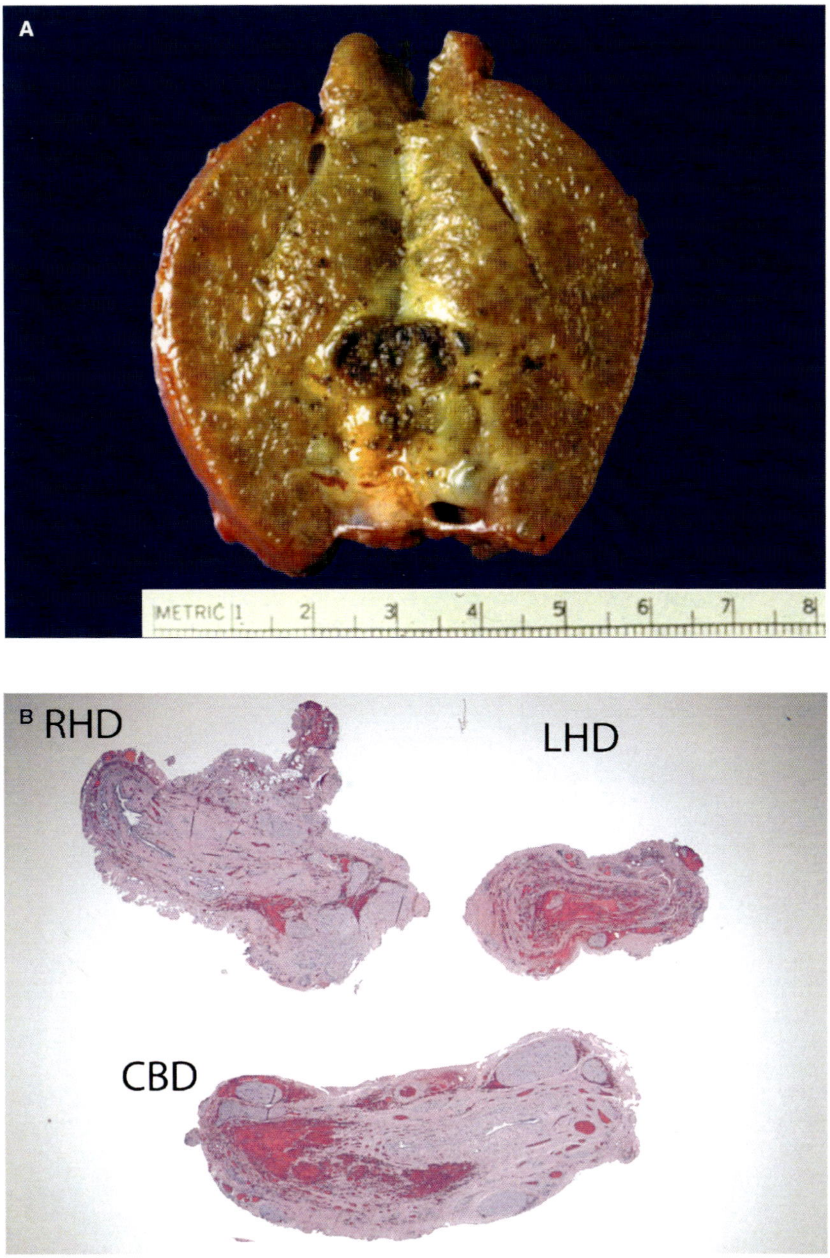

FIGURE 6-3

FIGURE 6-3 (A) Explanted cirrhotic liver due to extrahepatic BA, status post-Kasai procedure. The porta hepatis is extensively fibrotic with bile sludge in the anastomosed intestinal lumen. The remaining parenchyma exhibits bile-stained cirrhotic nodules. (B) Cross sections of the resected bile duct tree from another patient. As labeled, both the right hepatic duct (RHD) and the common bile duct (CBD) contain epithelium-lined ductal lumens, whereas the left hepatic duct (LHD) is completely obliterated leaving a fibrous cord.

(*continued*)

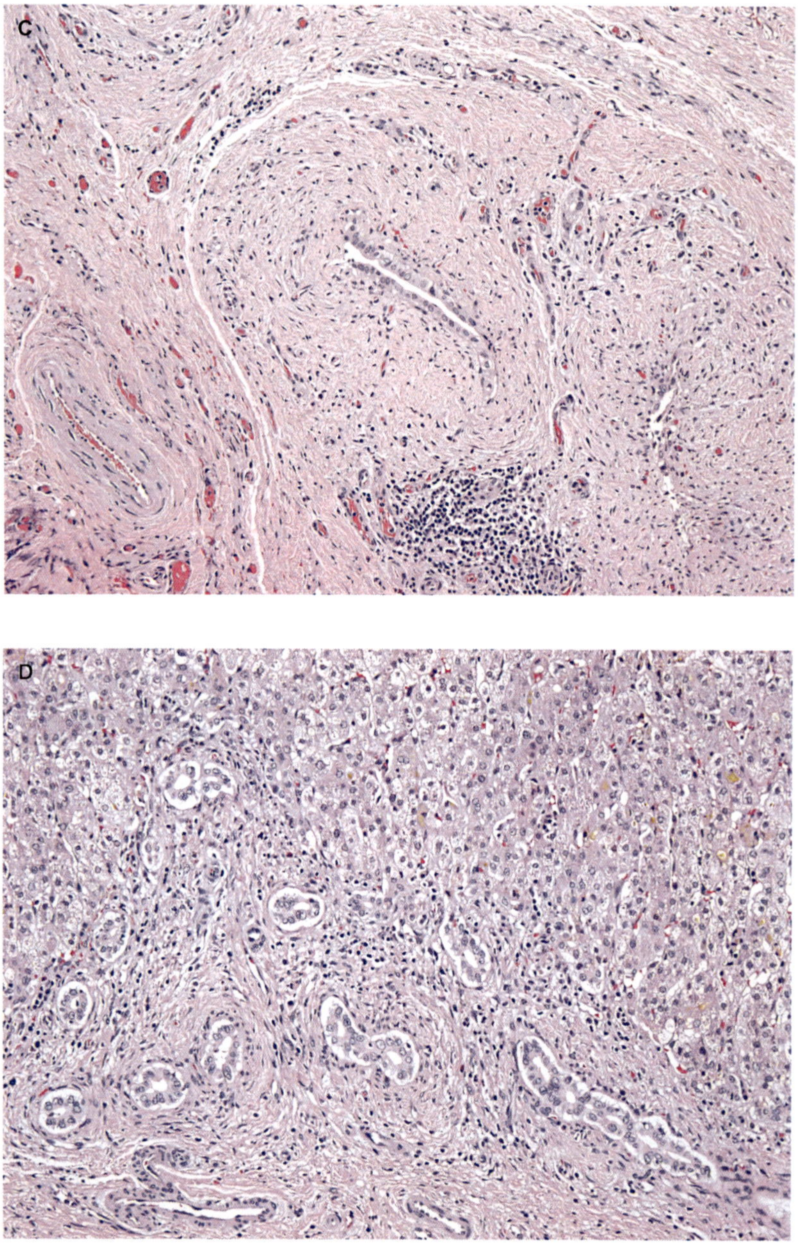

FIGURE 6-3

FIGURE 6-3 (C) A larger intrahepatic bile duct in the same liver as Figures 6-3B and 6-3D exhibits marked periductal "onion" skin type fibrosis, due to obstruction by BA. The ductal epithelium has started to show focal degeneration. Eventually these intrahepatic ducts will disappear as well, resulting in cirrhosis as seen in Figure 6-3A. (D) Intraoperative liver biopsy showing marked portal fibrosis, bile ductular proliferation, and canalicular cholestasis.

Liver Allograft Pathology

7

DONOR LIVER EVALUATION

PRESERVATION INJURY

ACUTE HUMORAL REJECTION

ACUTE CELLULAR REJECTION

CHRONIC REJECTION

GRAFT VERSUS HOST DISEASE (GVHD)

DE NOVO AUTOIMMUNE HEPATITIS

RECURRENT DISEASES

Donor Liver Evaluation

DEFINITION

Biopsy assessment of the donor liver for features related to long-term functioning of graft and patient survival

CLINICAL FEATURES

- For cadaver organ, frozen sections are performed when there are questionable factors for suitability of transplantation (i.e., extended donor criteria such as donors older than 60 years, steatotic graft).
- Macrovesicular steatosis increases susceptibility to preservation/reperfusion injury.
- For living donors, evaluation is achieved in permanent sections.

PATHOLOGIC FEATURES

- Features to evaluate: inflammation, fibrosis, necrosis; macrovesicular steatosis
- Macrovesicular steatosis (Figure 7-1A) greater than 30%: considered not suitable for transplant
- Distinction between macro- and microvesicular steatosis: fat droplets larger or smaller than the nuclear size of hepatocytes
- Microvesicular steatosis may be seen with warm ischemia, and does not adversely affect graft function.
- Necrosis greater than or equal to 10%: unacceptable
- Fibrosis greater than or equal to stage 2: unacceptable

DIFFERENTIAL DIAGNOSIS

- Frozen artifact (Figures 7-1B, C, D)

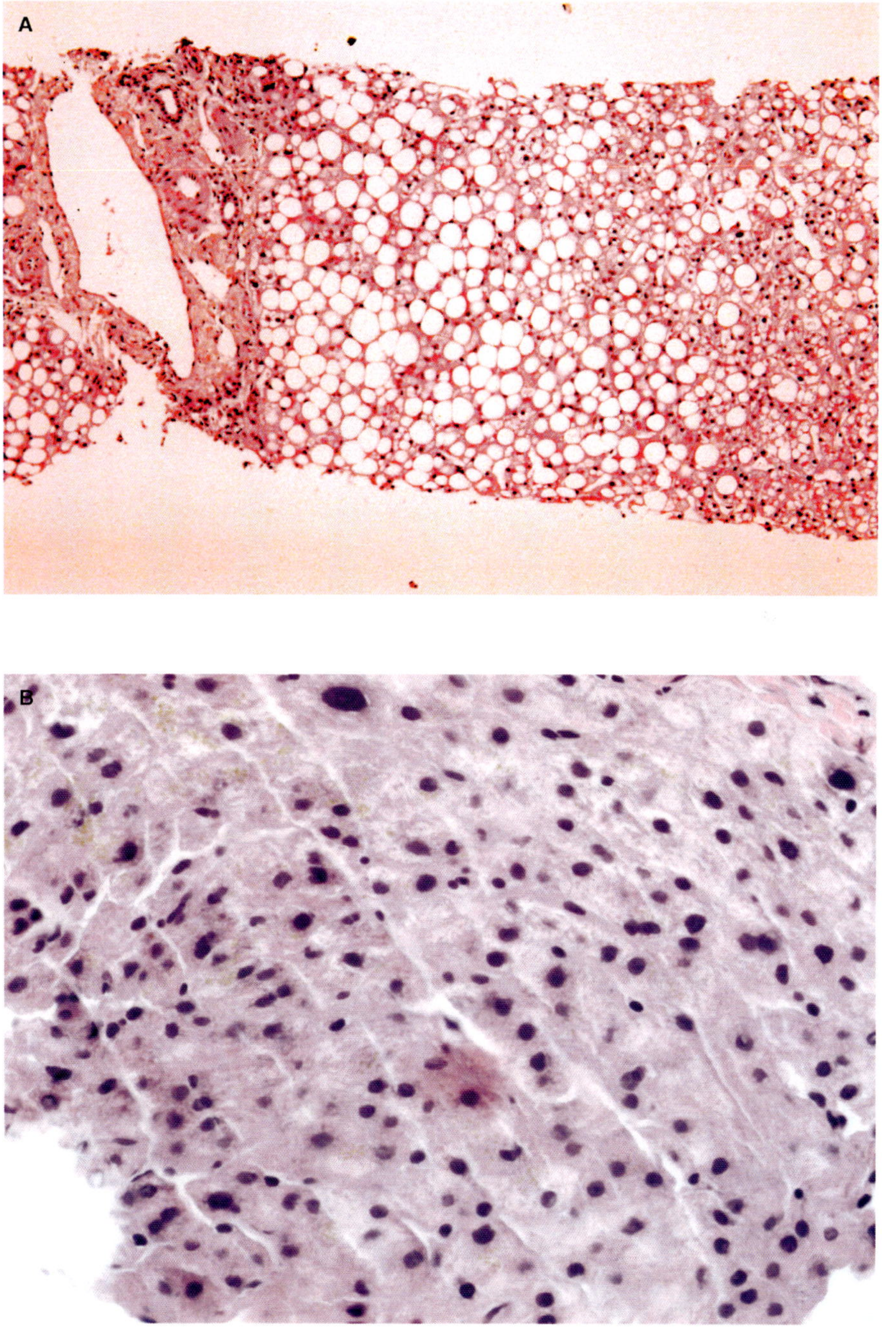

FIGURE 7-1

FIGURE 7-1 (A) Steatosis, not cytoplasmic round vacuoles with sharp edges. (B) Permanent section of the same specimen as in C and D. No steatosis.

(continued)

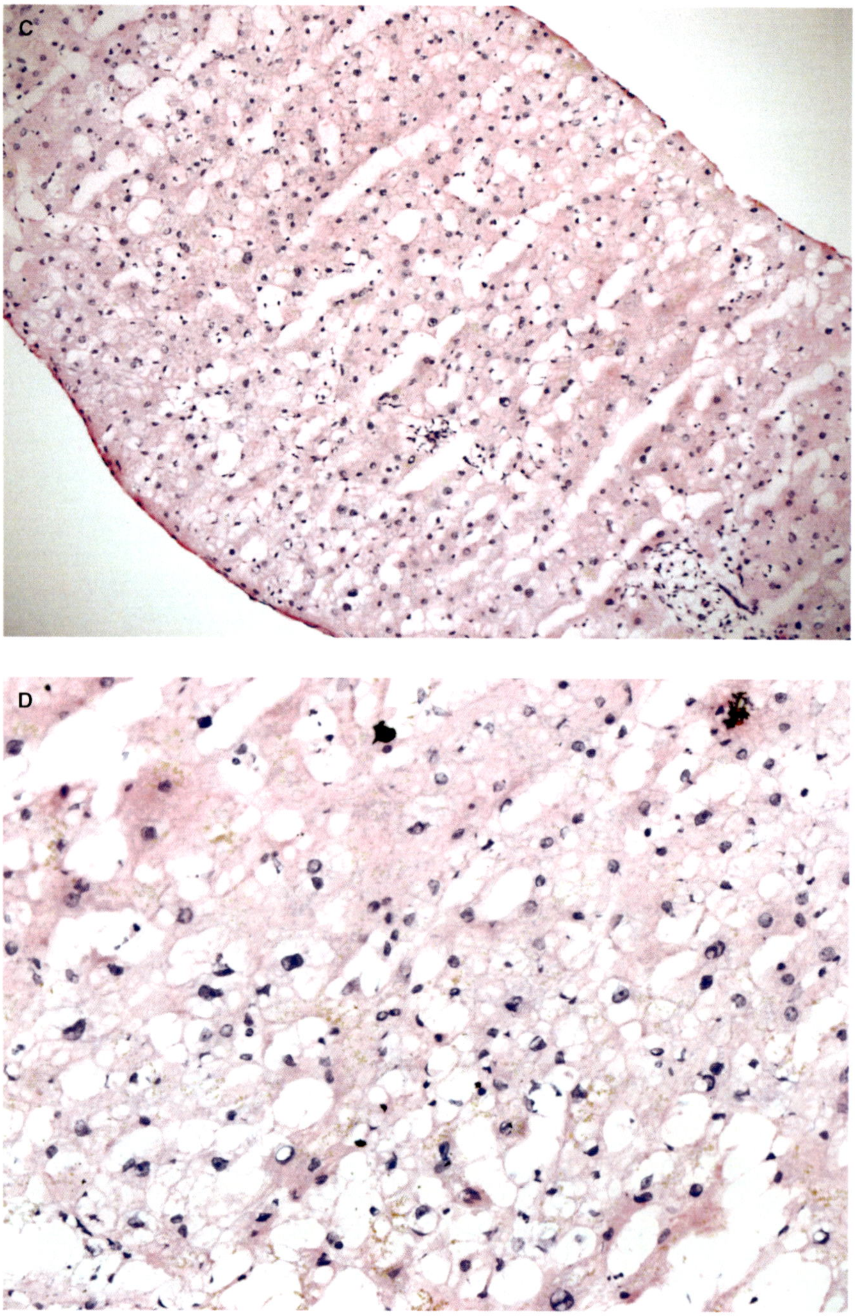

FIGURE 7-1

FIGURE 7-1 (C) Donor liver with frozen artifact. (D) At higher magnification, many irregular vacuoles that can be mistaken for fat droplets.

Preservation Injury

DEFINITION

Donor liver abnormalities present in peri-operative period (about 2 weeks after transplantation) that are related to harvest, transportation, and reperfusion and resolve spontaneously

CLINICAL FEATURES

- Donor risk factors: severe macrovesicular steatosis; donor death due to cardiac cause
- Poor bile production, persistent elevation of serum lactase, and elevation of transaminases after revascularization
- Two major types of injury: warm ischemia initiated during surgery or shock, and cold ischemia initiated during preservation
- Clinical resolution within 1 to 4 weeks

PATHOLOGIC FEATURES

- Canalicular cholestasis, balloon degeneration, or focal hepatocyte necrosis (Figures 7-2A, B)
- Histiocytes to phagocytic degenerative hepatocytes
- Baseline changes: minimal microvesicular steatosis, scattered acidophil bodies, or residual "surgical hepatitis"

DIFFERENTIAL DIAGNOSIS

- Antibody-mediated rejection
- Hepatic artery thrombosis

(*continued*)

Preservation Injury *(continued)*

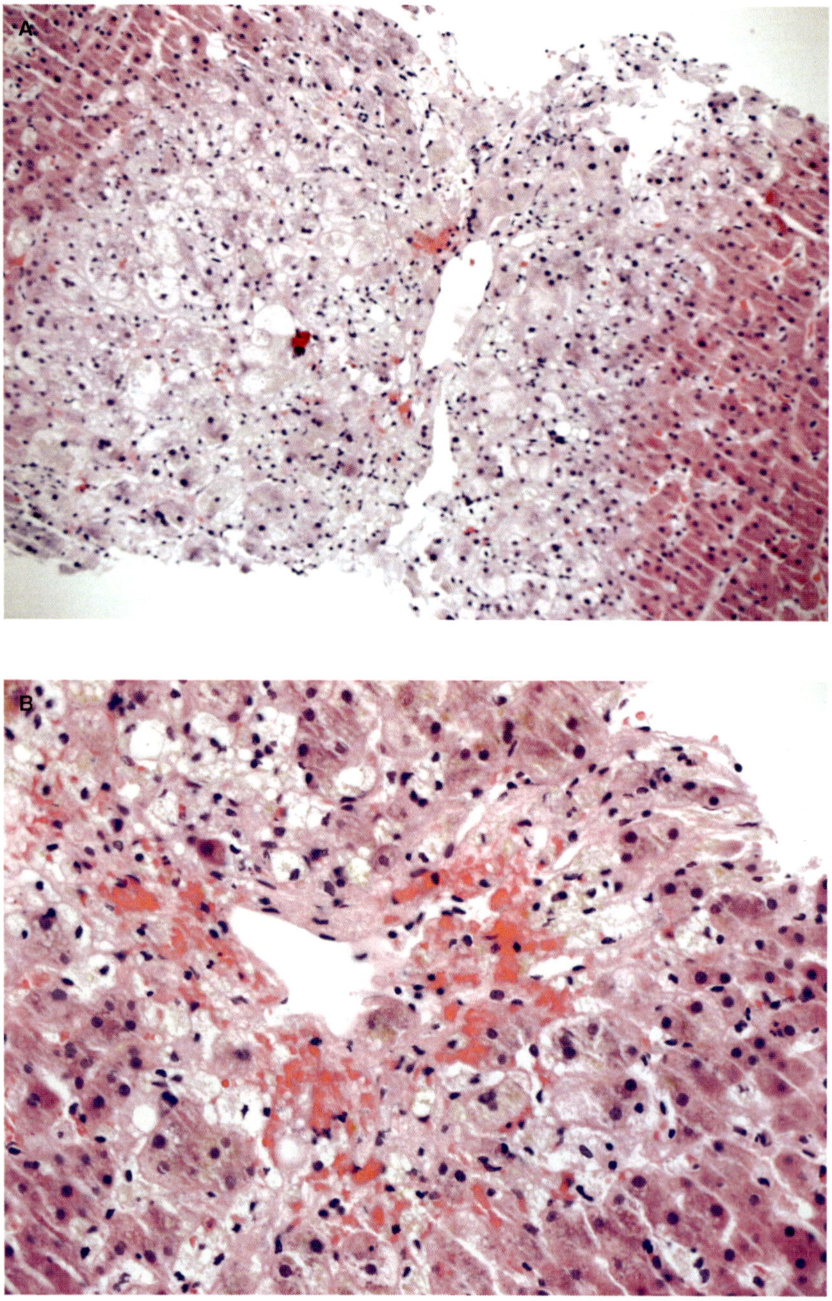

FIGURE 7-2

FIGURE 7-2 (A) Preservation injury. Zone 3 hepatocytes ballooning with pale appearance, and sharp demarcation from adjacent normal liver parenchyma. (B) Zone 3 necrosis, ballooning degeneration, cholestasis.

Acute Humoral Rejection

DEFINITION

Graft dysfunction mediated by antibody and complement occurring immediately or during the first week after transplantation. Antibodies include anti-histocompatibility complex, anti-ABO, and anti-endothelial

CLINICAL FEATURES

- Allograft swollen
- Slow or no bile production
- Coagulopathy
- Donor specific antibodies

HISTOLOGIC FINDINGS

- Sinusoidal congestion
- Hemorrhage and coagulative necrosis related to endothelial injury (severe cases) (Figures 7-3A, B, C)
- Portal edema, bile ductular proliferation, and neutrophils rich infiltrate resembling biliary obstruction (mild case)
- Immunohistochemical stain for C4d showing diffuse portal stroma positivity in more than 50% of portal tracts or sinusoids

DIFFERENTIAL DIAGNOSIS

- Preservation injury
- Biliary obstruction

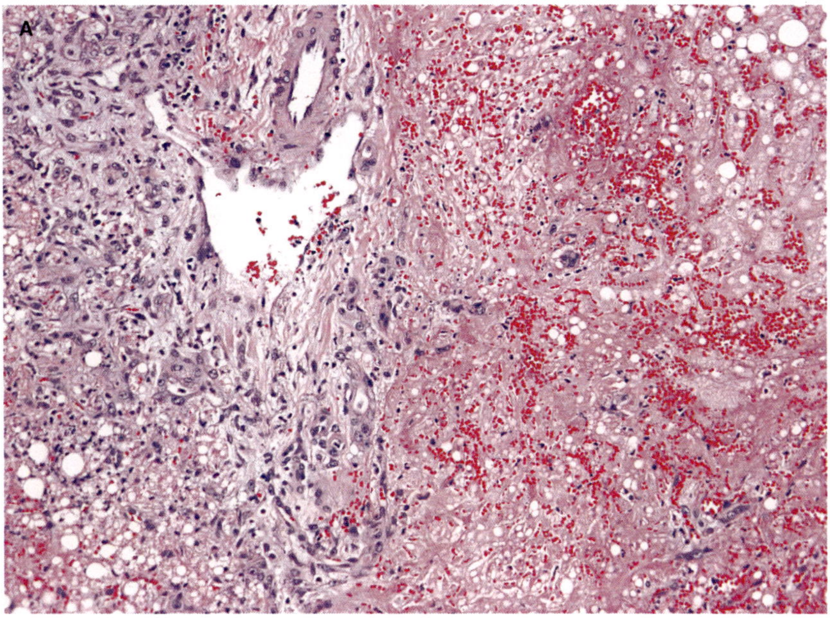

FIGURE 7-3

FIGURE 7-3 (A) Humoral rejection. Massive hepatocytic necrosis; portal tract with ductular proliferation, edema, and hemorrhage.

(*continued*)

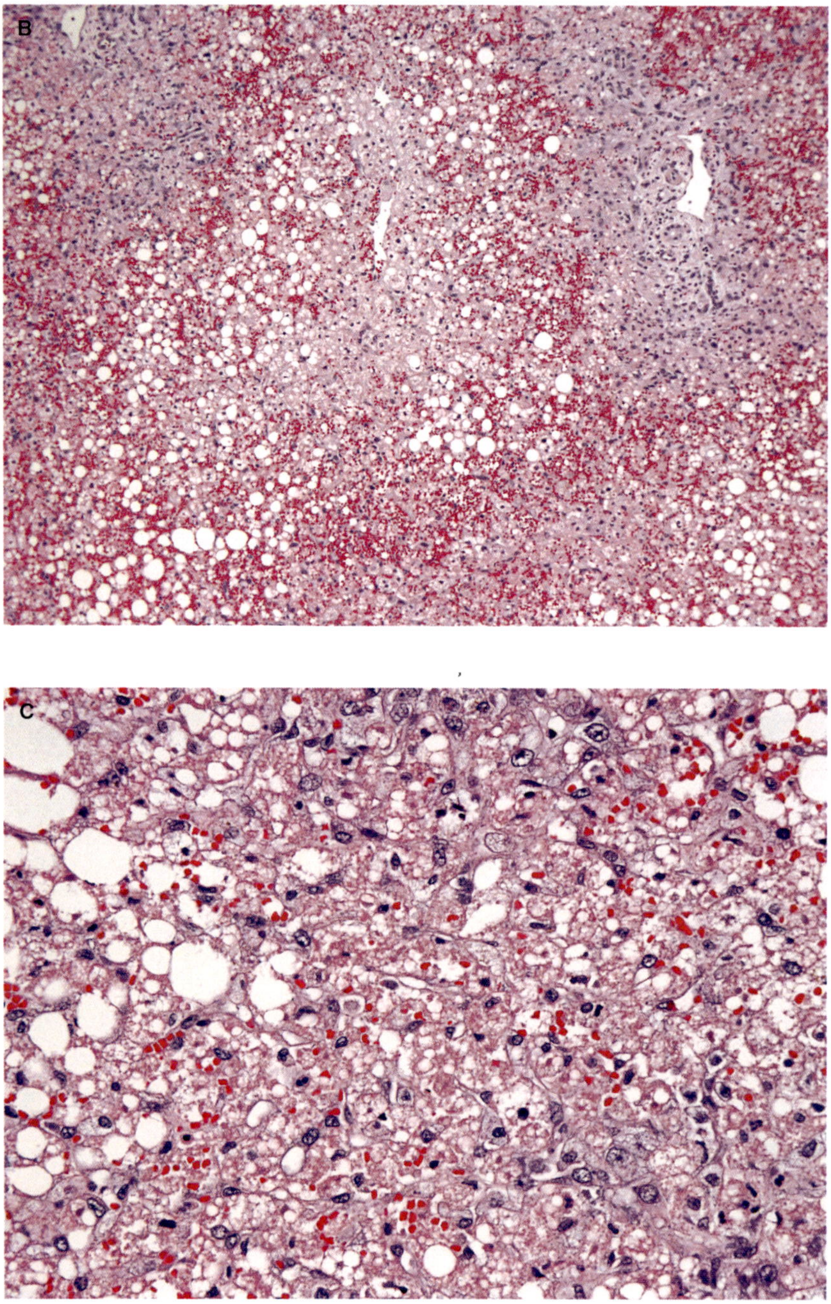

FIGURE 7-3

FIGURE 7-3 (B) Hemorrhage and coagulative necrosis mainly involving periportal zone, with steatosis. (C) Detailed view of coagulative necrosis.

Acute Cellular Rejection

DEFINITION

Allograft injury mediated by host lymphocytes preferentially targeting bile ducts, with associated liver function abnormalities

CLINICAL FEATURES

- Most occurring within 1 month after transplantation; however, mean time to first onset of acute rejection can be delayed to 100 later for patients who received pretransplant immunodepletion
- Increased risk: younger recipient age, older donor age, presence of immune dysregulation in recipient (autoimmune hepatitis [AIH], primary biliary cirrhosis, primary sclerosing cholangitis), HLA-DR mismatch, extended cold ischemic time
- Late-onset acute rejection may be due to decreased immunosuppression or noncompliance.
- Usually asymptomatic
- Mild nonspecific elevation of serum AST and ALT, alkaline phosphatase, bilirubin
- Peripheral leukocytosis with eosinophilia
- Bile drainage from T-tube decreases with altered color and texture (thinner material)

PATHOLOGIC FEATURES

- Mixed portal inflammatory infiltrate composed predominantly of lymphocytes with few plasma cells, neutrophils and eosinophils (Figure 7-4A)
- Bile duct injury with pleomorphic biliary epithelial nuclei with lymphocytic cholangitis, uneven nuclear spacing, cytoplasmic eosinophilia, and vacuolation (Figure 7-4B)
- Endothelialitis (undermining of vascular endothelium by lymphocytes with "lifting up" of endothelium) involving portal or central venule
- So-called central-type form may present with only endothelialitis; this histologic finding alone is suggestive, but not diagnostic, of acute rejection
- Late-onset acute rejection may resemble a chronic hepatitis

DIFFERENTIAL DIAGNOSIS

Preservation injury
Recurrent viral hepatitis C
Recurrent AIH

Special note: Liver allografts are very "forgiving" compared with other allografts: they can recover from most rejection-related injury without fibrosis. On another hand, over-treatment with immunosuppression may significantly worsen hepatitis or even trigger *fibrosing cholestatic hepatitis* (FCH). Therefore, when biopsies show features of concurrent acute rejection and recurrent hepatitis C, assigning "blame" of tissue injury should be leaning toward the latter, to avoid unnecessary even harmful increase in immunosuppression.

(*continued*)

Acute Cellular Rejection *(continued)*

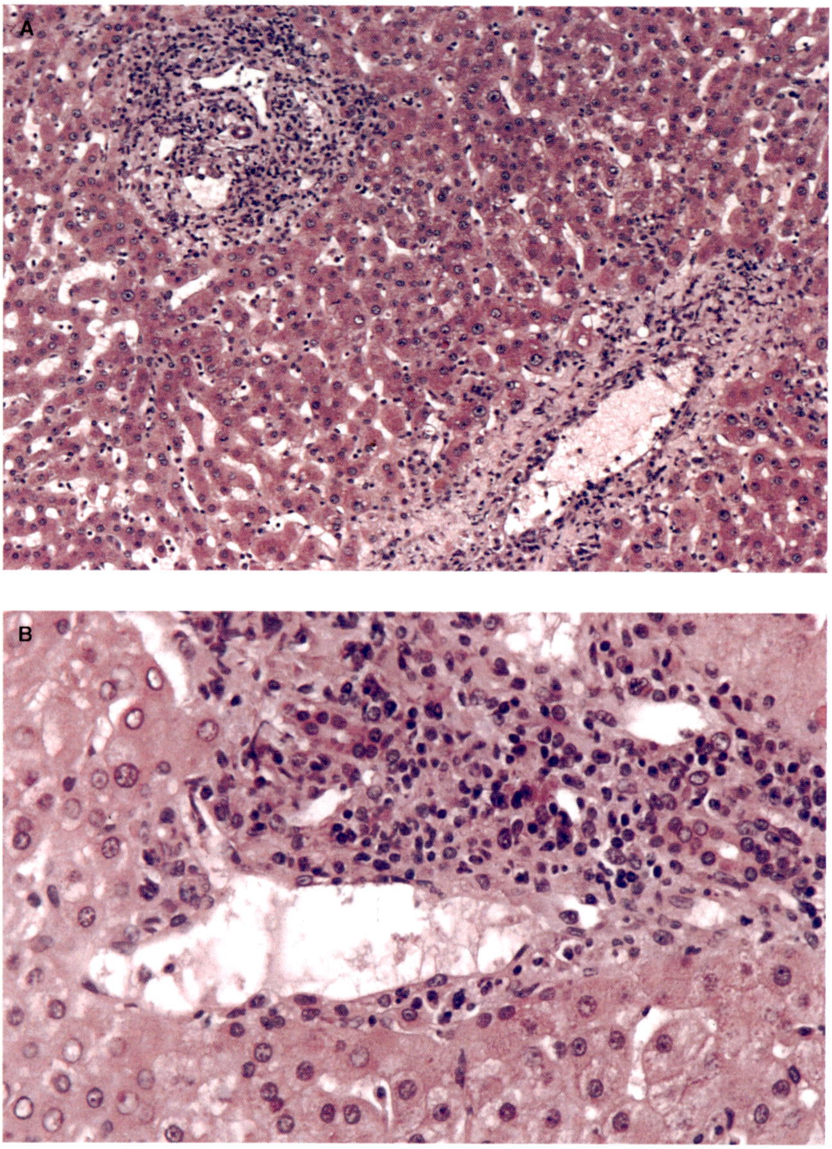

FIGURE 7-4

FIGURE 7-4 (A) Moderate acute cellular rejection. A portal tract (upper left) with mixed inflammatory cellular infiltration, bile duct injury, and endotheliitis of the portal vein. Marked endotheliitis is also evident involving a terminal hepatic venule (lower left corner). (B) Higher power view of a portal tract with rejection type inflammation, with lymphocytes lifting endothelium of the portal vein. The bile duct becomes obscured with active lymphocytic infiltration.

Chronic Rejection

DEFINITION

Immune mediated damage to the allograft associated with potentially irreversible injury to bile ducts, arteries, and veins

CLINICAL FEATURES

- Usually do not occur within 60 days of transplantation
- Repeated or prolonged episodes of acute rejection common
- May occur without episode of acute rejection
- Jaundice and elevated liver enzyme with progressive cholestatic pattern

HISTOLOGIC FEATURES

- Ductopenia (loss of small bile ducts greater than 50%) (Figures 7-5A, B)
- Degenerative changes in remaining bile ducts
- Obliterative arteriopathy with foamy cells (Figure 7-5C)
- Zone 3 hepatocytes necrosis (Figure 7-5D)

DIFFERENTIAL DIAGNOSIS

- Ischemic cholangiopathy
- Recurrent primary biliary cirrhosis (PBC) or primary sclerosing cholangitis (PSC)
- Biliary obstruction

(*continued*)

Chronic Rejection *(continued)*

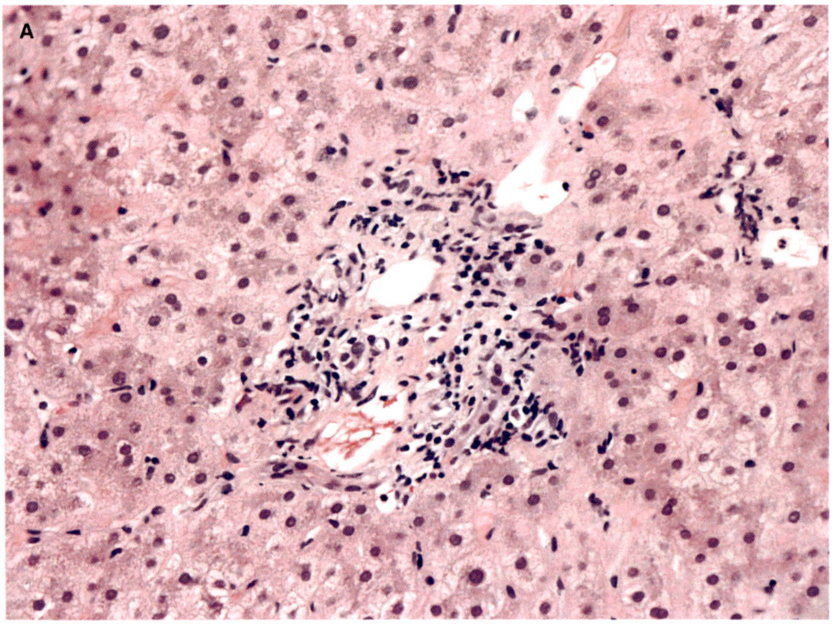

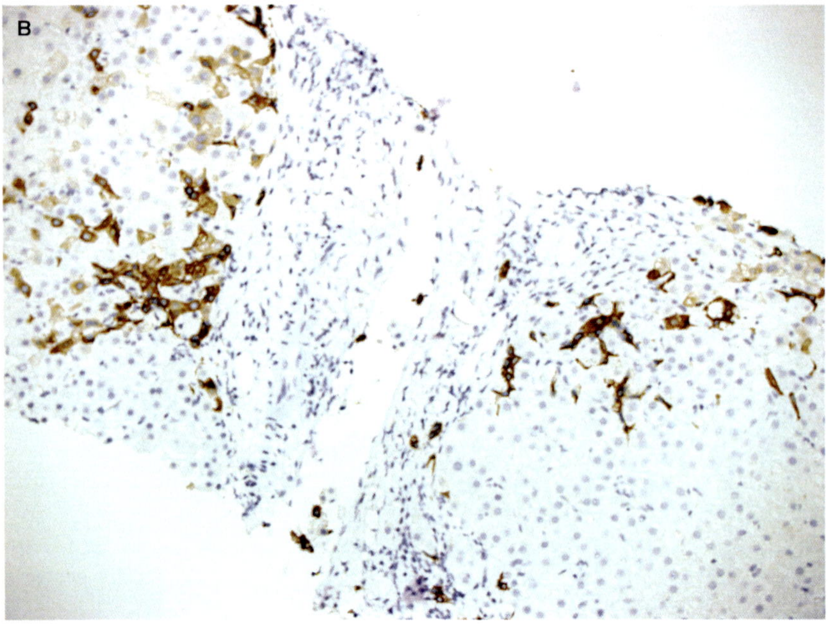

FIGURE 7-5

FIGURE 7-5 (A) Chronic rejection. A portal tract with bile duct loss. (B) Immunohistochemical stain for CK7 highlights hepatic progenitor cells but no interlobular bile ducts in this portal tract.

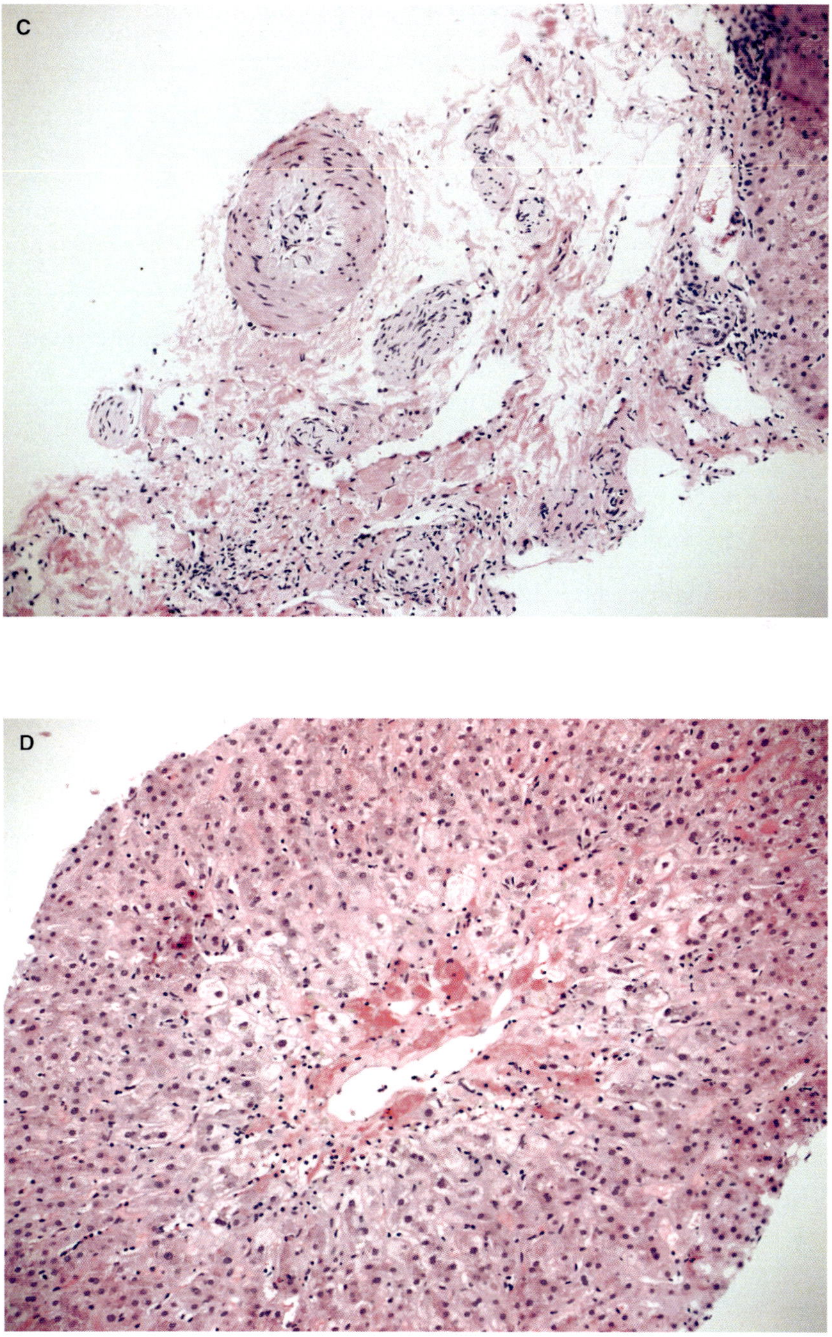

FIGURE 7-5

FIGURE 7-5 (C) Obliterative arteriopathy with foamy cell. (D) Centrilobular hepatocyte dropout.

Graft Versus Host Disease (GVHD)

DEFINITION

Immune-mediated injury of host tissue by allogeneic donor T lymphocytes

CLINICAL FEATURES

- Most commonly seen after allogeneic bone marrow or stem cell transplantation; rarely with solid organ transplantation
- Jaundice, elevated liver enzyme with cholestatic pattern
- Hepatomegaly
- Acute GVHD less than 100 days posttransplant; chronic GVHD greater than 100 days posttransplant
- Acute GVHD affects skin, gastrointestinal tracts, and liver
- Chronic GVHD in addition may affect musculoskeletal, oral and ocular area

HISTOLOGIC FEATURES

- Bile duct injury: nuclear pleomorphism, disarray, intraepithelial lymphocytes, ductopenia (Figures 7-6A, B)
- Acidophil bodies (Figure 7-6C)
- Rare histology: endotheliitis, lobular inflammation, acute hepatitis

DIFFERENTIAL DIAGNOSIS

- Drug-induced liver injury

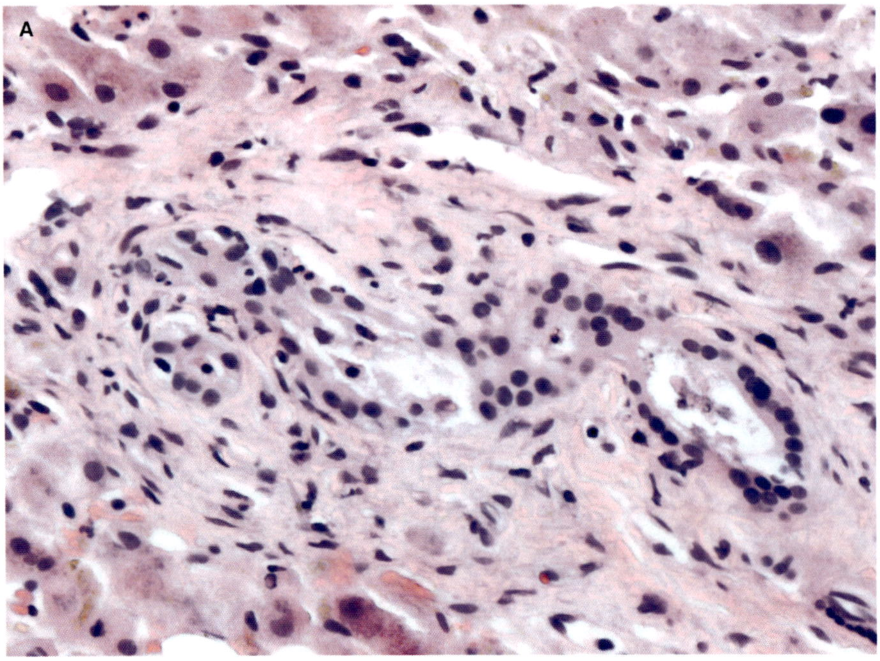

FIGURE 7-6

FIGURE 7-6 (A) Acute GVHD. Bile duct epithelium is unevenly spaced and intraepithelial lymphocytes are noted.

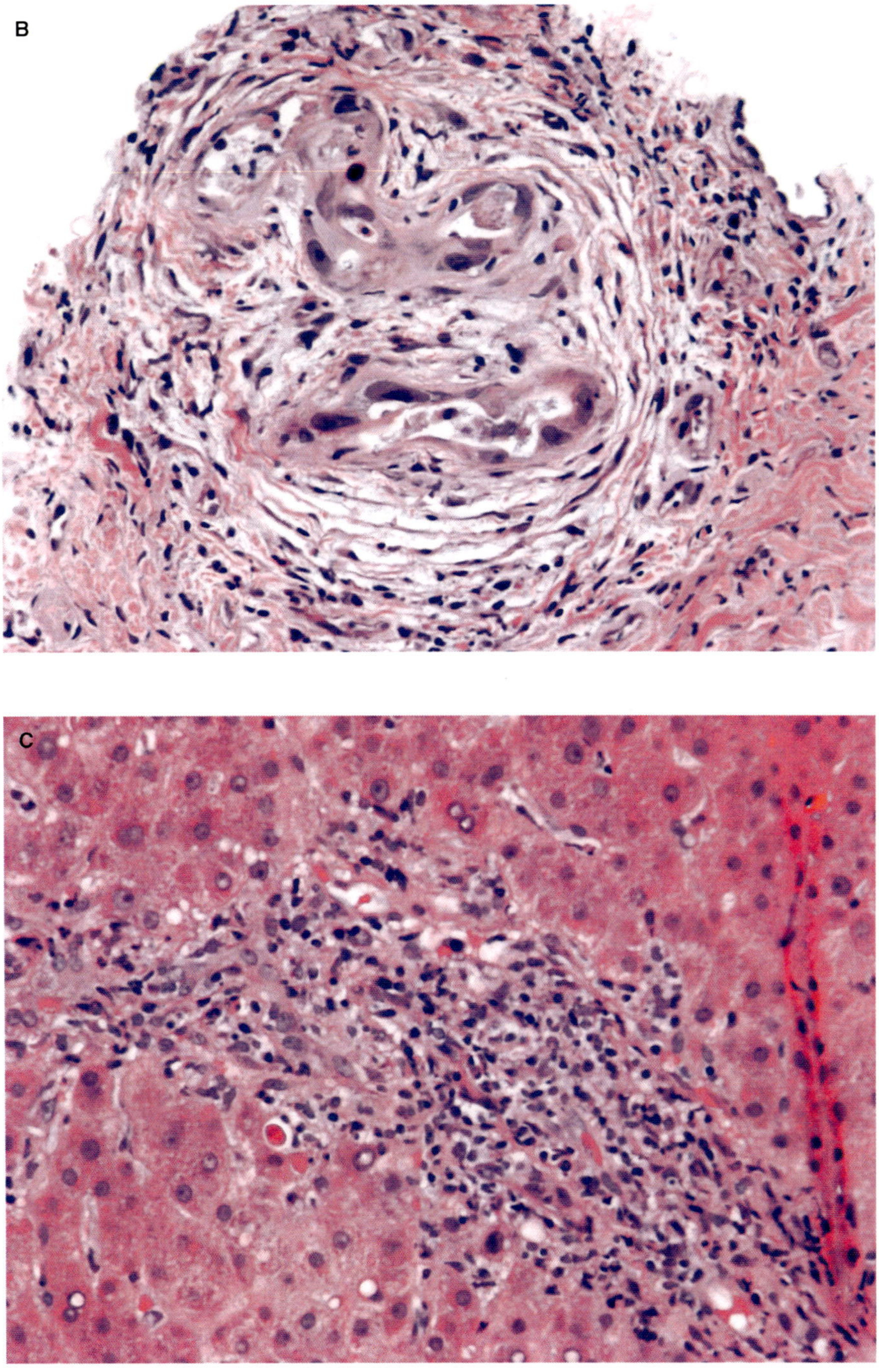

FIGURE 7-6

FIGURE 7-6 (B) Bile duct injury characterized by nuclear pleomorphism. (C) Chronic GVHD. Bile duct loss and acidophil bodies.

De Novo Autoimmune Hepatitis

DEFINITION

Allograft dysfunction resembling AIH developed in patients with no history of pretransplant AIH.

CLINICAL FEATURES

- Biochemical and serological results same as AIH
- Autoantibodies present in approximately 50% to 70% of cases
- More common in children (6%–10%) than in adults (2%–3%)
- More common in the patients with previous PBC or PSC
- Occurs between 2 and 5 years posttransplantation
- May represent a specific form of rejection (injury directed toward hepatocytes rather than bile ducts or endothelium)

HISTOLOGIC FEATURES

- Histology similar to classic AIH (prominent plasma cells with interface hepatitis) (Figure 7-7A)
- Severe cases showing bridging or confluent necrosis (Figure 7-7B)
- Lobular necroinflammation with perivenular inflammation

DIFFERENTIAL DIAGNOSIS

- Recurrent chronic hepatitis C

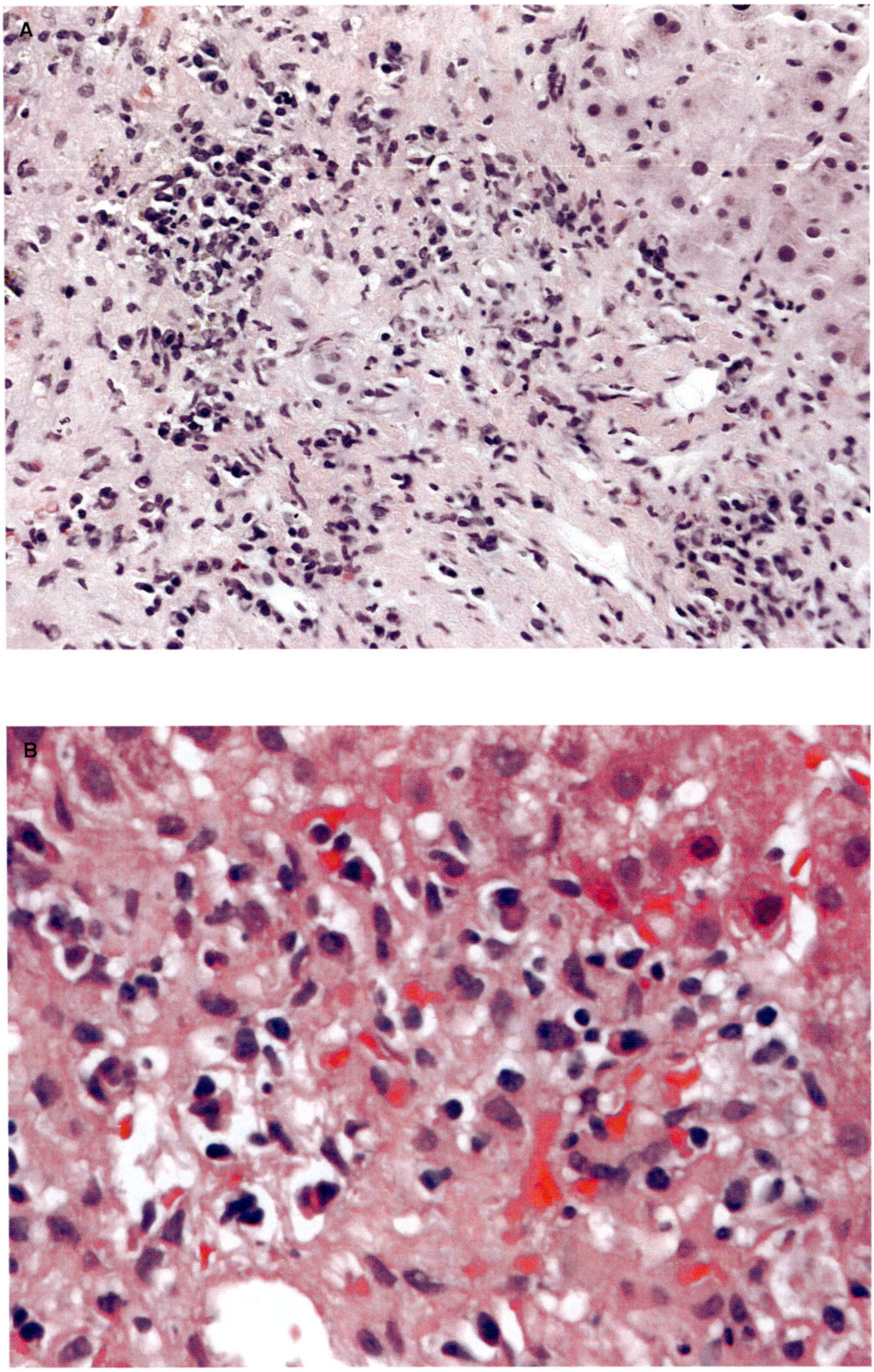

FIGURE 7-7

FIGURE 7-7 (A) De novo AIH. Lymphoplasmacytic infiltration with interface activity. (B) Central perivenulitis. Zone 3 hepatocytes necrosis associated with lymphoplasmacytic infiltrate.

Recurrent Diseases

DEFINITION

Recurrence of the original disease for which the transplant was performed

CLINICAL FEATURES

- Infectious diseases: hepatitis B virus (HBV) and hepatitis C virus (HCV) will universally re-infect the new liver
- Immune-mediated diseases (PBC, PSC, AIH, and overlap disease): commonly recur (20%–30% by 5 years after transplantation)
- Hepatocellular carcinoma: recurrence depending on tumor volume. Cases within the Milan criteria (one lesion smaller than 5 cm, up to three lesions smaller than 3 cm, no extrahepatic manifestations, no vascular invasion) are less likely to recur
- Toxic and metabolic disease (alcohol and nonalcoholic fatty liver disease [NAFLD]): rate of alcoholic liver disease relapse difficult to document precisely (13%–50% by 5 years); NAFLD recur 25% to 100% by 5 years
- Hepatic-based metabolic disease (alpha-1-antitrypsin deficiency, Wilson's disease, tyrosinemia): liver transplant curable (no recurrence)
- Nonhepatic-based metabolic disease (hereditary hemochromatosis, cystic fibrosis, Niemann–Pick disease): recurs, but transplantation improves survival

HISTOLOGIC FEATURES

- Histology similar to the original disease, but may overlap with other transplant-related complication (i.e., recurrent chronic hepatitis C and acute cellular rejection) (Figures 7-8A, B, C)
- Immunosuppressive therapy modifies disease severity (HCV behaves more aggressive, AIH behaves less aggressive)
- Distinction between recurrent hepatitis C and acute rejection most common problem, but identifying the prevailing process (acute rejection versus recurrent hepatitis C) more important than absolute differentiation

DIFFERENTIAL DIAGNOSIS

- Acute cellular rejection
- Biliary obstruction

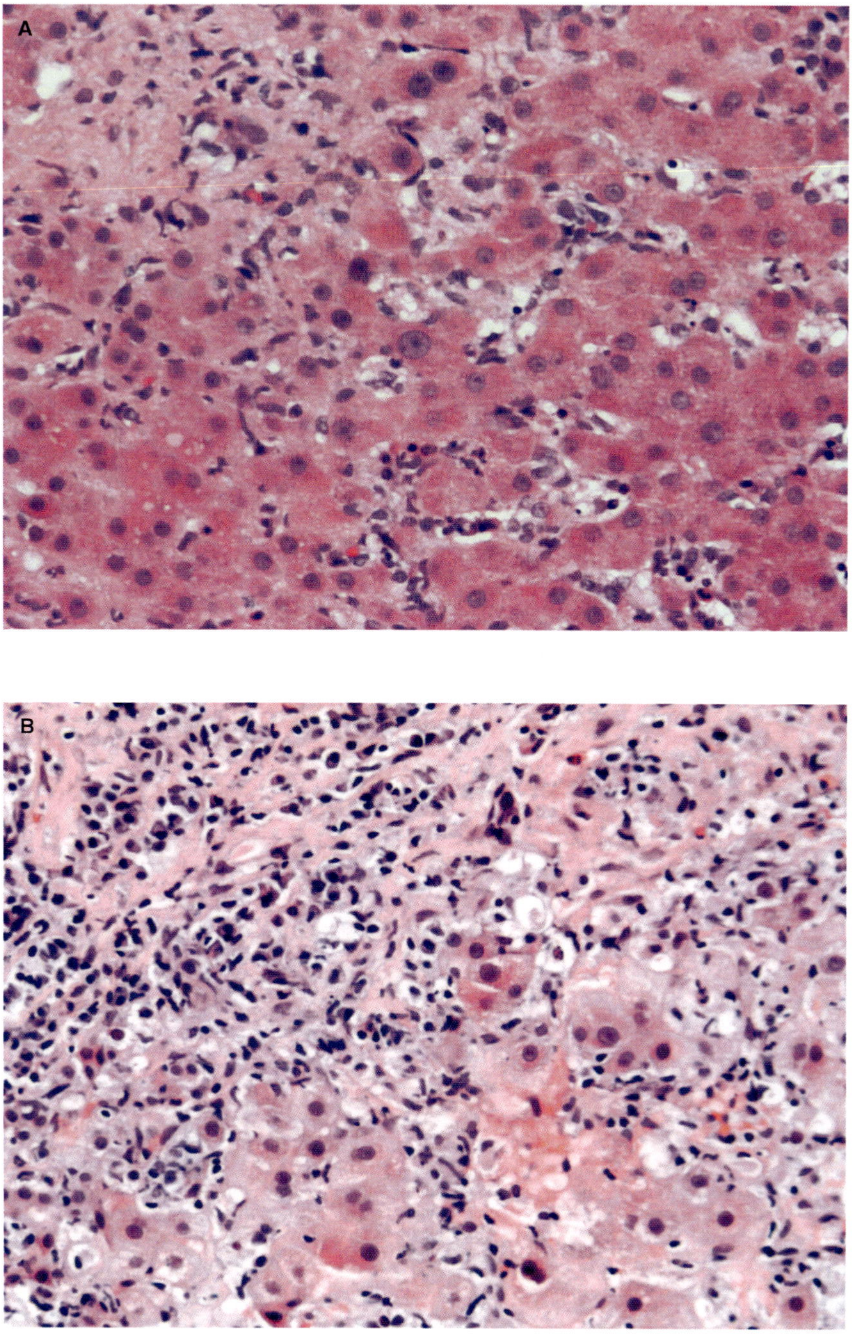

FIGURE 7-8

FIGURE 7-8 (A) Recurrent HCV, 1 month posttransplantation. Lobular disarray, Kupffer cell hypertrophy, and mild sinusoidal lymphocytosis are present. (B) Recurrent AIH. Prominent plasma cell infiltration with interface activity.

(*continued*)

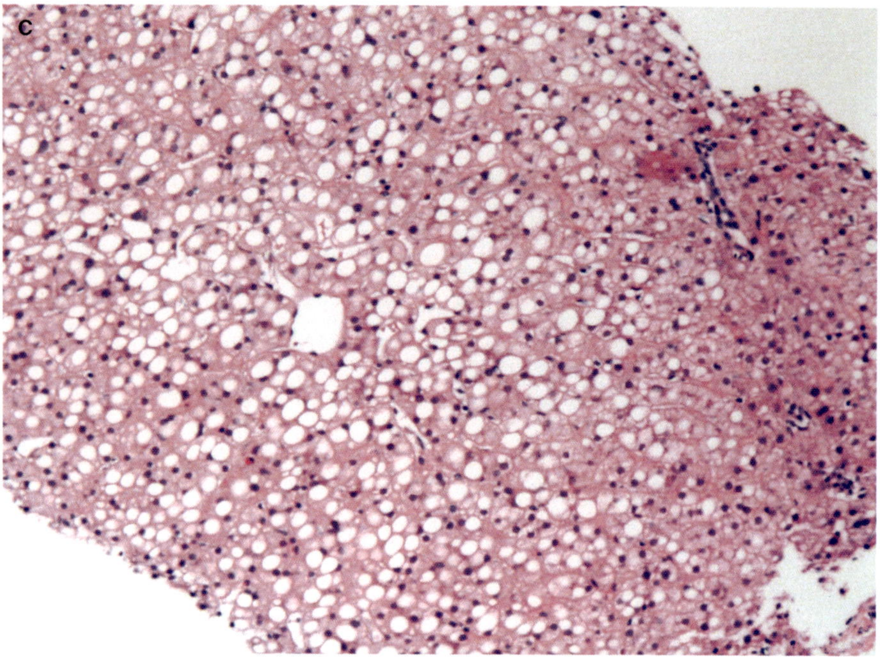

FIGURE 7-8

FIGURE 7-8 (C) Recurrent NAFLD, 6 month posttransplantation. Macrovesicular steatosis is seen involving 70% of the parenchyma, with rare balloon cell degeneration.

8

Liver Involvement in Other Systemic Diseases

Lymphoma Involving Liver

DEFINITION

Both secondary involvement by disseminated lymphoma and primary lymphoma occur in the liver (the latter, hepatosplenic lymphoma, is very rare).

CLINICAL FEATURES

- Primary lymphoma occurs in patients of all ages
- Some associated with viral hepatitis, HIV
- Posttransplant lymphoproliferative disorder (PTLD) associated with Epstein-Barr virus (EBV)
- Abdominal pain, swelling, fever, or liver mass
- Some present with acute liver failure

PATHOLOGIC FEATURES

- Diffuse large B-cell lymphoma most common, with nodular and diffuse infiltration by large atypical lymphocytes (Figures 8-1A, B)
- Many other types also seen, including small lymphocytic B-cell lymphoma, Burkitt lymphoma, mucosa-associated lymphoid tissue (MALT) lymphoma; chronic lymphocytic leukemia shows mostly portal expansion by uniform small lymphocytes (Figure 8-1C)
- Primary hepatosplenic lymphoma: prominent sinusoidal infiltration by clusters of atypical lymphocytes expressing T cell markers (Figure 8-1D)
- Hodgkin's lymphoma involving the liver exhibits similar histologic features as in other sites

DIFFERENTIAL DIAGNOSIS

- Chronic hepatitis C (portal lymphoid nodules) versus small B-cell lymphoma
- Infectious mononucleosis versus large B-cell or hepatosplenic lymphoma
- Inflammatory pseudotumor versus Hodgkin's lymphoma

A

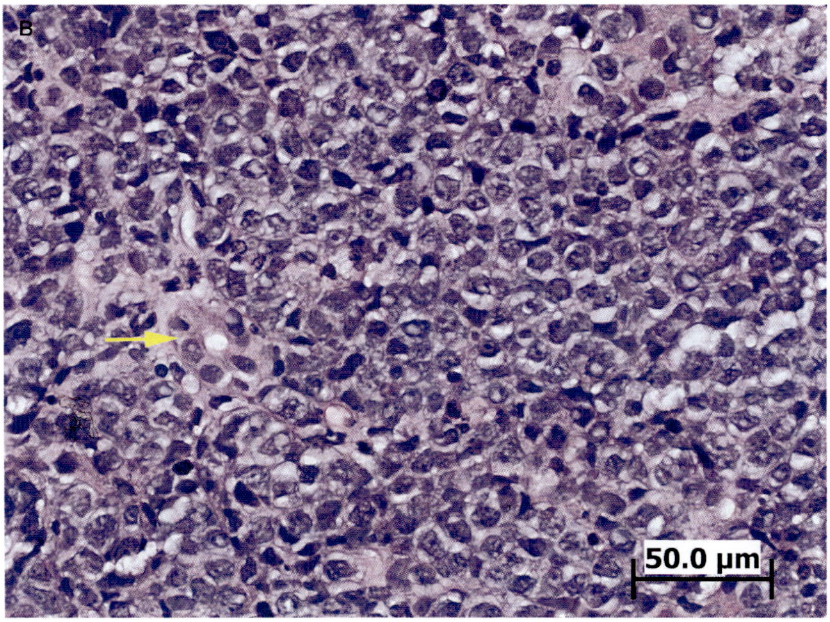

FIGURE 8-1

FIGURE 8-1 (A) Diffuse large B-cell lymphoma. Prominent infiltration involves the portal tracts and lobular parenchyma. (B) Diffuse large B-cell lymphoma. This field depicts the infiltration of large lymphocytes, which expands the portal tract, with an "entrapped" bile duct (arrow).

(*continued*)

Lymphoma Involving Liver *(continued)*

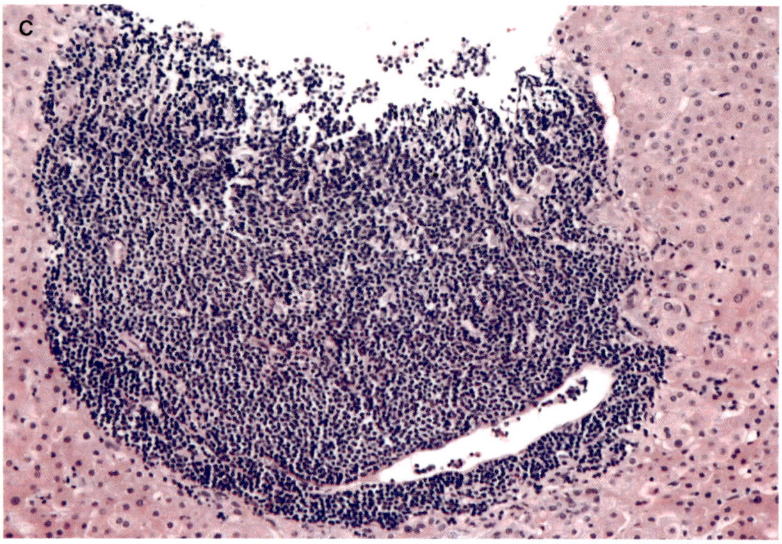

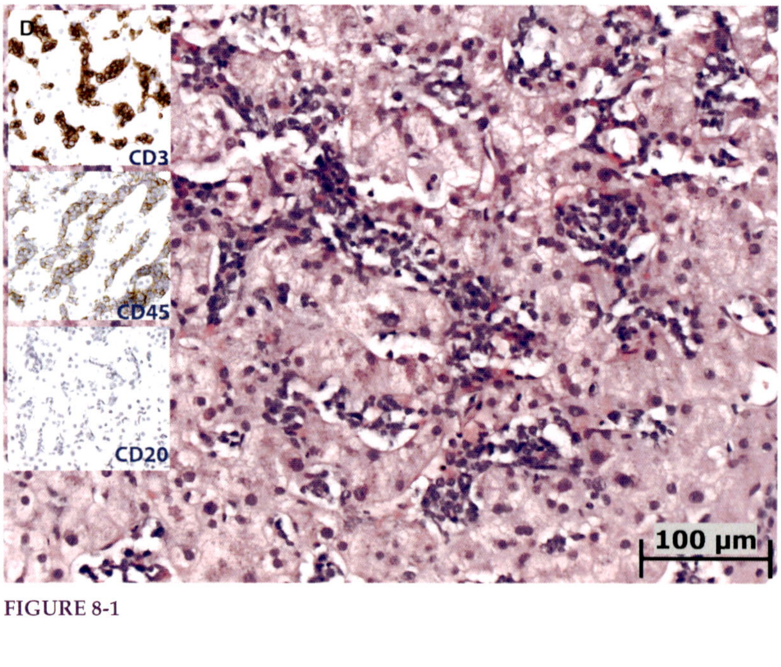

FIGURE 8-1

FIGURE 8-1 (C) Hepatic involvement by chronic lymphocytic leukemia: nodular infiltration expanding a portal tract. (D) Hepatosplenic T-cell lymphoma. There is prominent sinusoidal infiltration by clusters of atypical T lymphocytes.

Systemic Lupus Erythematosus

DEFINITION

Chronic liver diseases occur in about 2.5% to 5% of patients with systemic lupus erythematosus (SLE), which may lead to significant mortality from hepatic failure. Chronic liver diseases of other etiologies should be excluded.

CLINICAL FEATURES

- Persistent elevation of serum transaminases (in about 10% of SLE patients)
- Jaundice
- Serum antinuclear antibody
- Anti-phospholipid antibody (syndrome)

PATHOLOGIC FEATURES

- The pathologic changes are essentially nonspecific, including macrovesicular steatosis (Figure 8-2A) and mild portal or periportal lymphocytic infiltration (Figure 8-2B).
- Several other conditions have rarely been reported in SLE patients: chronic hepatitis with or without cirrhosis, primary biliary cirrhosis, nodular regenerative hyperplasia, peliosis hepatis, and arteritis with hepatic infarction.
- Macrovesicular steatosis may be related to corticosteroid therapy in some patients.

DIFFERENTIAL DIAGNOSIS

- Autoimmune hepatitis

(*continued*)

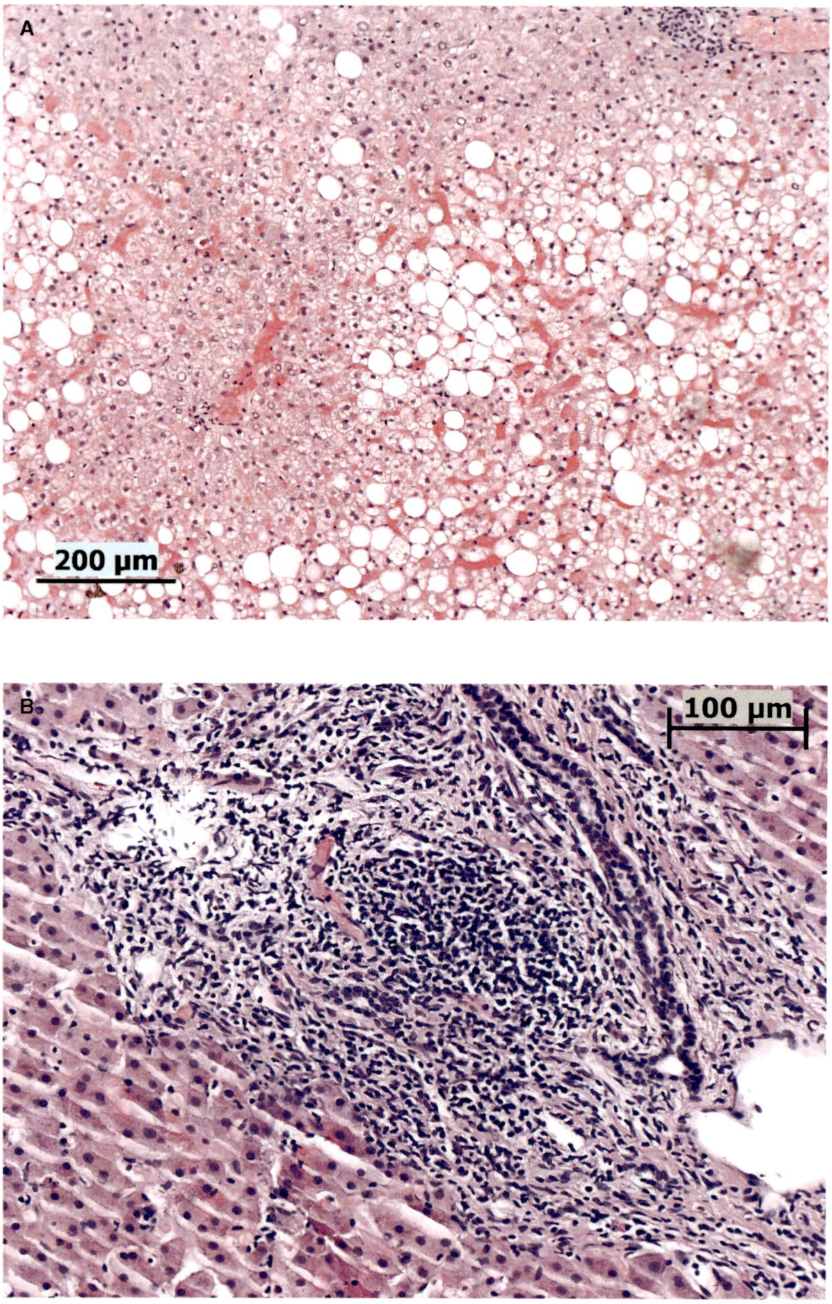

FIGURE 8-2

FIGURE 8-2 (A) Mild macrovesicular steatosis. (B) Mild portal infiltration by mostly lymphocytes, without significant injury to the layer of hepatocytes bordering the portal tract ("limiting plate").

9

Benign Epithelial Nodules and Tumors

FOCAL NODULAR HYPERPLASIA

HEPATIC ADENOMA

NODULAR REGENERATIVE HYPERPLASIA

Focal Nodular Hyperplasia

DEFINITION

A benign, nonneoplastic hepatocellular mass that arises in a non-cirrhotic background, typically in young women, and is characterized by hepatocyte hyperplasia and focal fibrosis

CLINICAL FEATURES

- Usually in patients in their third to fourth decades of life
- Male:female ratio = 1:5
- May be asymptomatic, or present with abdominal pain, weight loss, weakness, fever, or abdominal mass (only rarely with hemorrhage)
- Believed to arise as a hyperplastic growth response to altered blood flow caused by a preexisting "spider-like" arterial malformation
- May occur as part of a syndrome including multiple focal nodular hyperplasia (FNH), hepatic hemangioma, berry aneurysm, meningioma, astrocytoma, telangiectasia of the brain, dysplastic systemic arteries, and portal vein atresia

PATHOLOGIC FEATURES

- Usually solitary; multiple in 20% to 30% of cases
- Well-circumscribed, firm, tan-brown nodular mass with a central scar, often paler than surrounding liver (Figure 9-1A)
- Microscopically, sheets of bland hepatocytes arranged in nodules with incomplete fibrovascular septa radiating from the central scar ("focal cirrhosis") (Figure 9-1B)
- Hepatocellular cords two to three cell layers in thickness (Figure 9-1C)
- No normal portal tracts within the lesion (Figures 9-1B–D)
- Fibrovascular septa composed of large muscular blood vessels accompanied by proliferating bile ductules (Figure 9-1B, C)
- Immunohistochemical stain for glutamine synthetase displays a characteristic geographic map pattern

DIFFERENTIAL DIAGNOSIS

- Hepatic adenoma (HA), particularly the inflammatory type
- Nodular regenerative hyperplasia (NRH)

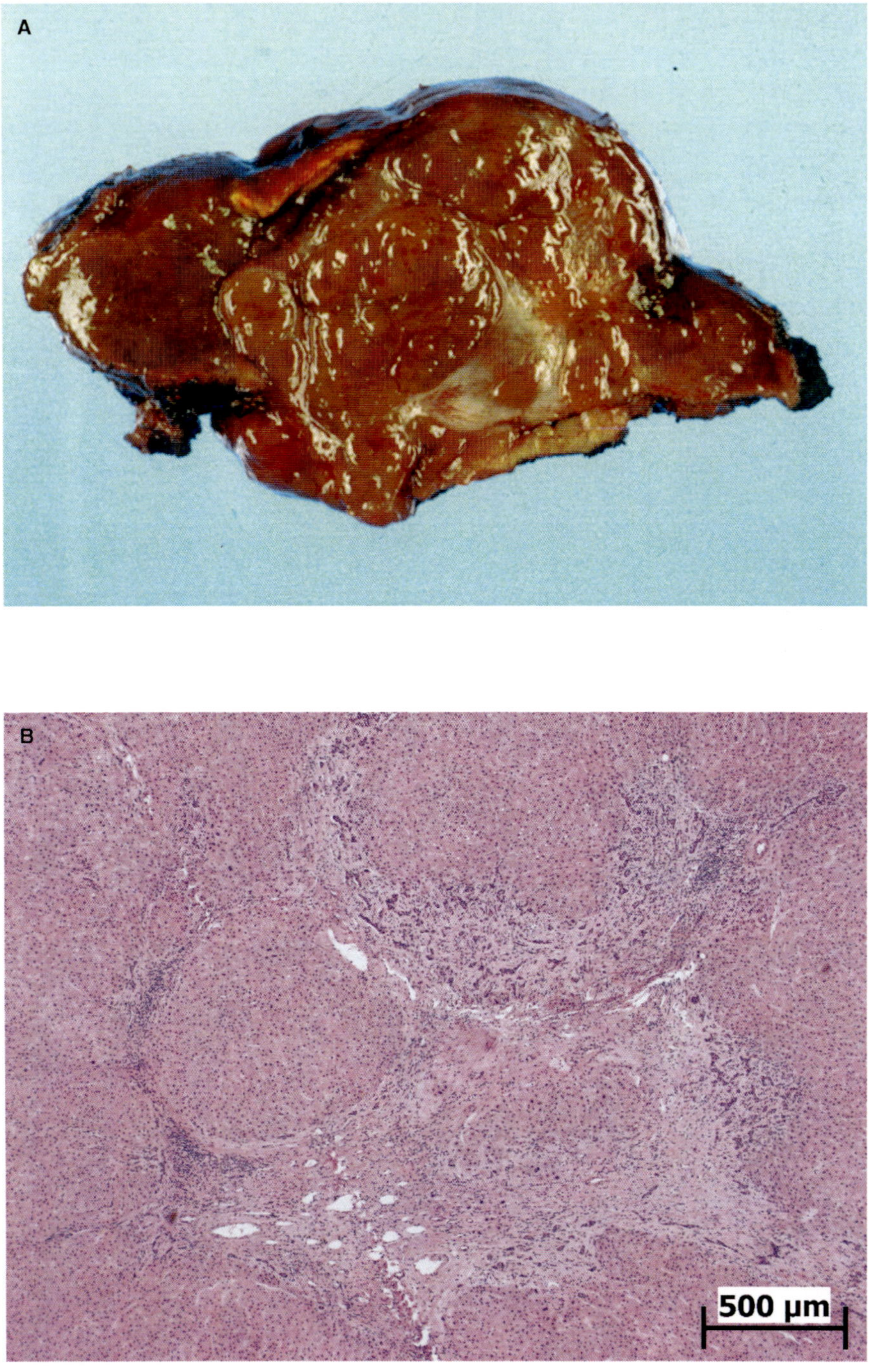

FIGURE 9-1

FIGURE 9-1 (A) FNH, with a central scar. (B) FNH. Small nodules and incomplete fibrous septa, with focal peri-nodular ductular proliferation.

(*continued*)

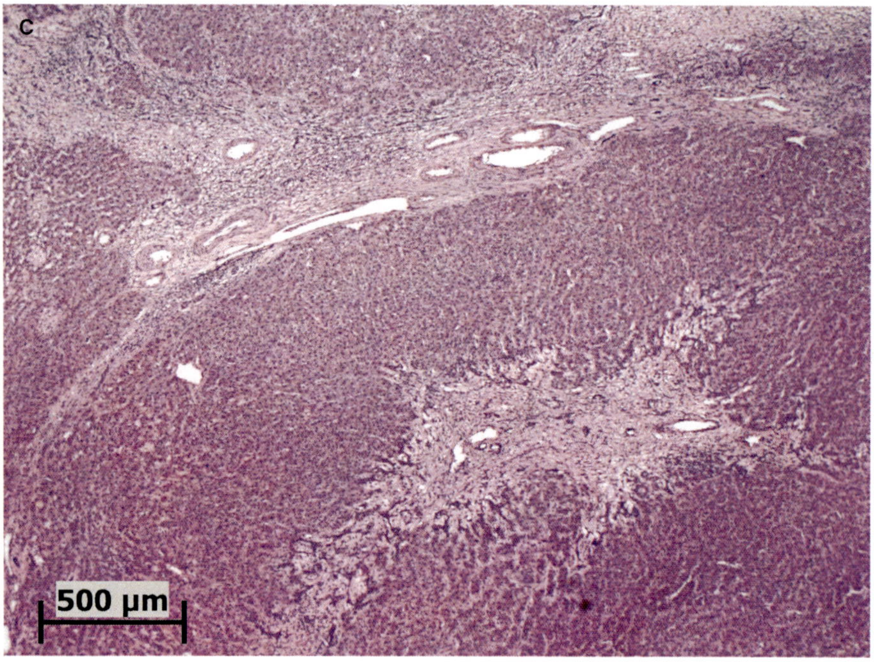

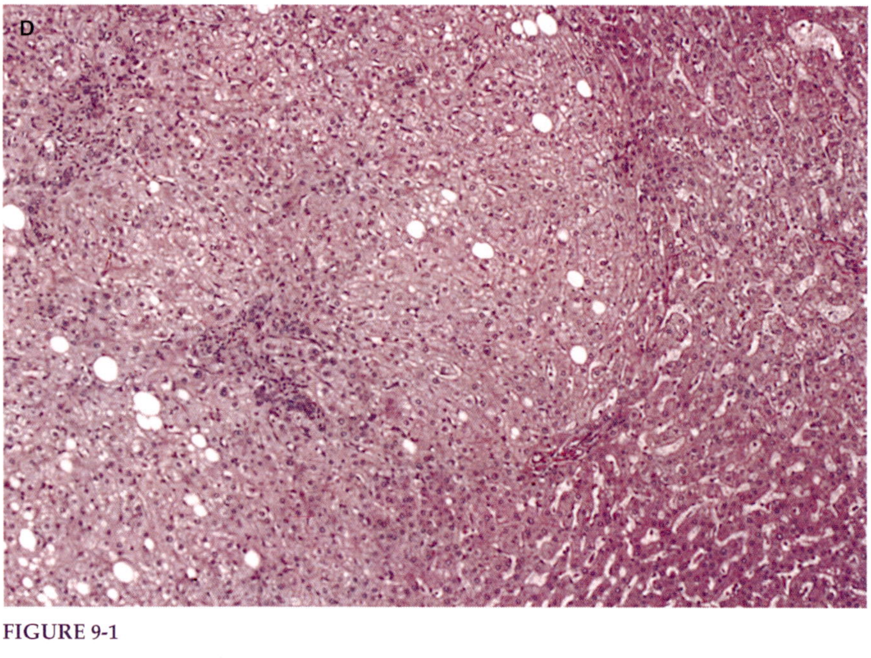

FIGURE 9-1

FIGURE 9-1 (C) Large thick-walled blood vessels are evident. (D) Distinct junction between FNH (left) and normal parenchyma (right).

Hepatic Adenoma

DEFINITION

Benign hepatocellular neoplasm that arises in a non-cirrhotic liver, usually in young women; also known as hepatocellular adenoma (HCA) or liver cell adenoma; malignant transformation in 6% to 10%

CLINICAL FEATURES

- Usually occurs in the third to fourth decades of life
- Male:female ratio = 1:15
- Associated with oral contraceptive use, diabetes mellitus, glycogen storage diseases, galactosemia, tyrosinemia
- Presents with abdominal mass, pain, nausea, or intra-abdominal bleeding

PATHOLOGIC FEATURES

- Solitary or multiple
- Solid, bulging, grossly well-circumscribed mass in a background of normal liver; demarcation from surrounding parenchyma sometimes inconspicuous (Figure 9-2A)
- Histologically, the borders of the mass are indistinct, fading imperceptibly into the surrounding hepatic parenchyma (Figure 9-2B)
- Composed of sheets of bland hepatocytes without intervening portal tracts but containing large muscular arterioles; hepatocellular cords two to three cell layers in thickness; may have steatosis or Mallory-Denk bodies in some cases (Figures 9-2B–D)
- Intratumoral sinusoidal dilatation or peliosis common (Figures 9-1B and C)
- Subtypes proposed: (1) inflammatory; (2) hepatocyte nuclear factor (HNF)-1a activated; (3) beta-catenin activated, and (4) unclassified

DIFFERENTIAL DIAGNOSIS

- FNH
- NRH
- Well-differentiated hepatocellular carcinoma

(*continued*)

Hepatic Adenoma *(continued)*

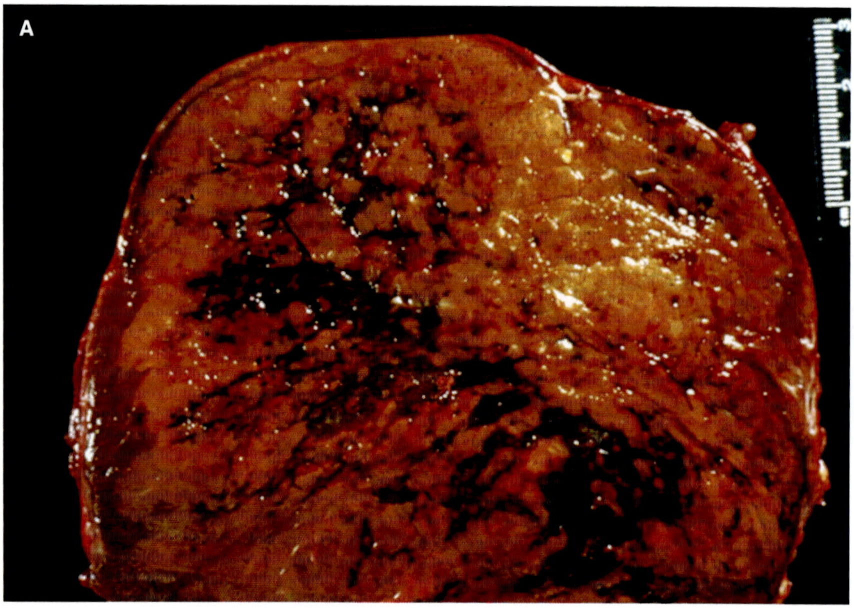

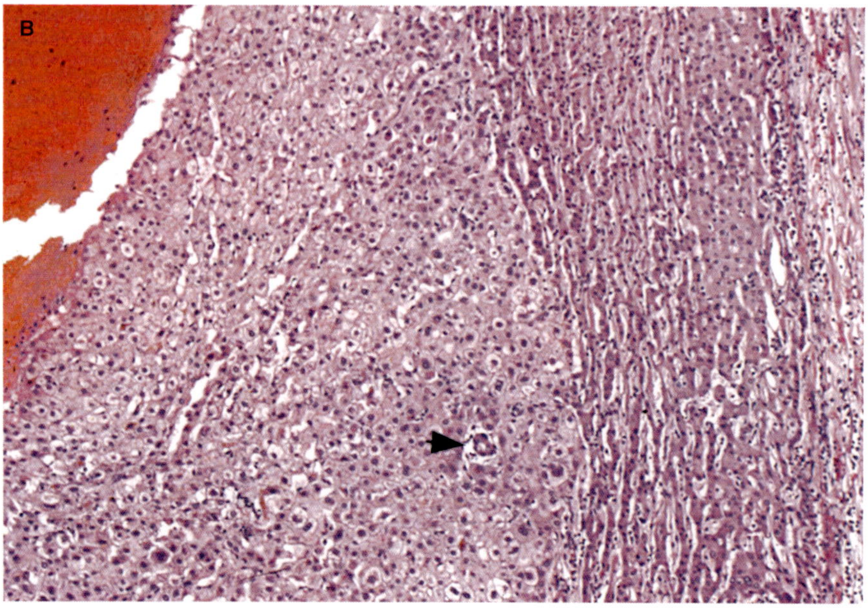

FIGURE 9-2

FIGURE 9-2 (A) A large HA, with variegated cut surface and prominent peliosis. Note the red-tan rim of normal parenchyma on the left edge. (B) HA (left) "pushing" into the adjacent parenchyma that appears atrophic. Note a "naked" arterial (arrowhead), and a "blood lake" on the left upper edge.

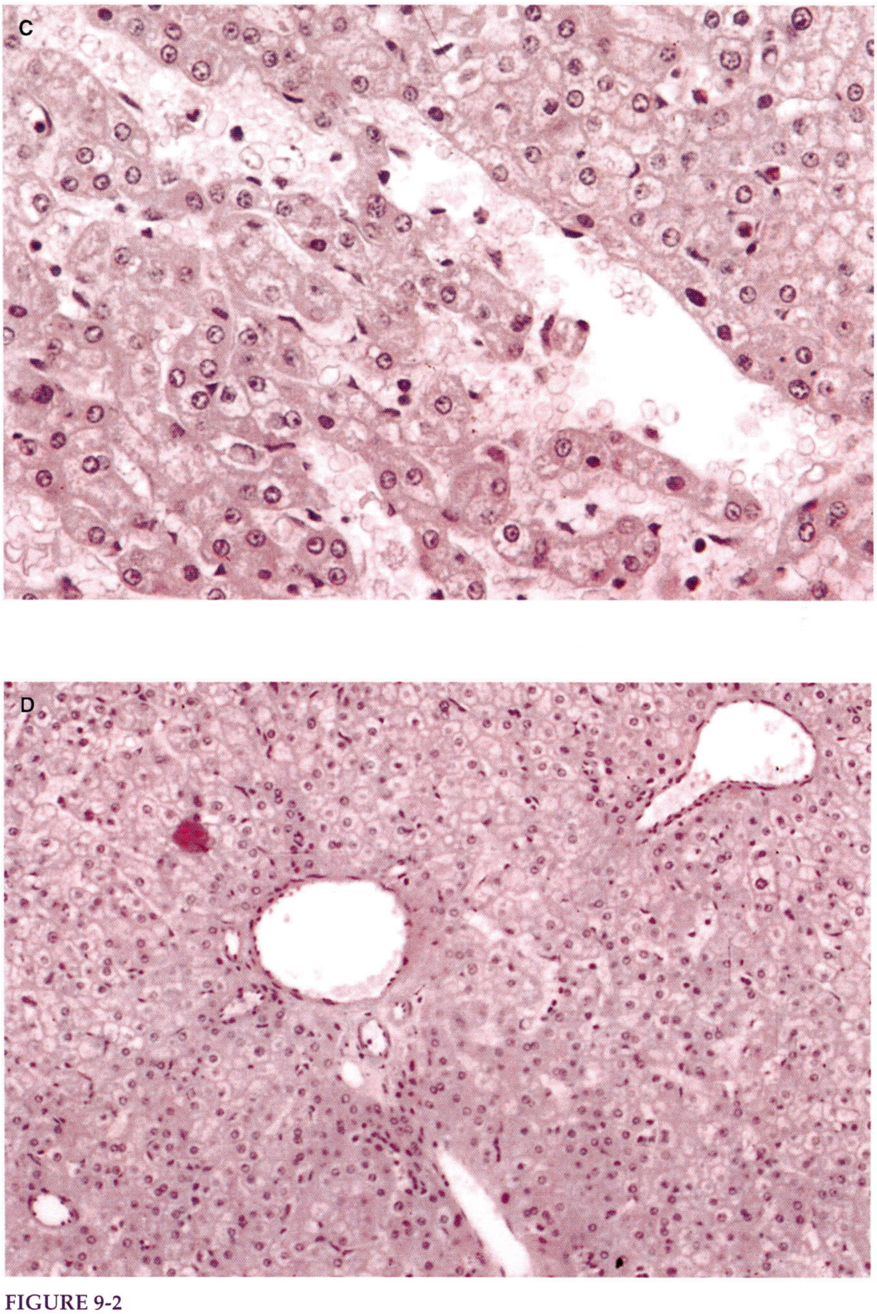

FIGURE 9-2

FIGURE 9-2 (C) Large and small intercellular "slits" characterize the intratumoral peliosis, which gives rise to the grossly hemorrhagic appearance. Note the lack of endothelial lining. (D) Areas resembling a portal tract can be seen, but with lack of bile ducts.

Nodular Regenerative Hyperplasia

DEFINITION

Transformation of hepatic parenchyma into diffuse small regenerative nodules (1–3 mm) with essentially no fibrosis

CLINICAL FEATURES

- Occurs in the background of other diseases: rheumatologic disorders, polycythemia vera, chronic leukemia, lymphoma; or may be associated with drugs (azathioprine, etc.)
- Nodular formation likely due to alteration in blood flow resulting from obliteration of small portal veins or damage to sinusoids
- Symptoms: portal hypertension

HISTOLOGIC FEATURES

- Vague parenchymal nodules (Figures 9-3A, B)
- Variation in size of hepatocytes due to unevenly distributed blood flow (Figure 9-3C)
- Sinusoidal dilatation focally
- Little or no fibrosis (Figure 9-3D)

DIFFERENTIAL DIAGNOSIS

- Cirrhosis
- Focal nodular hyperplasia

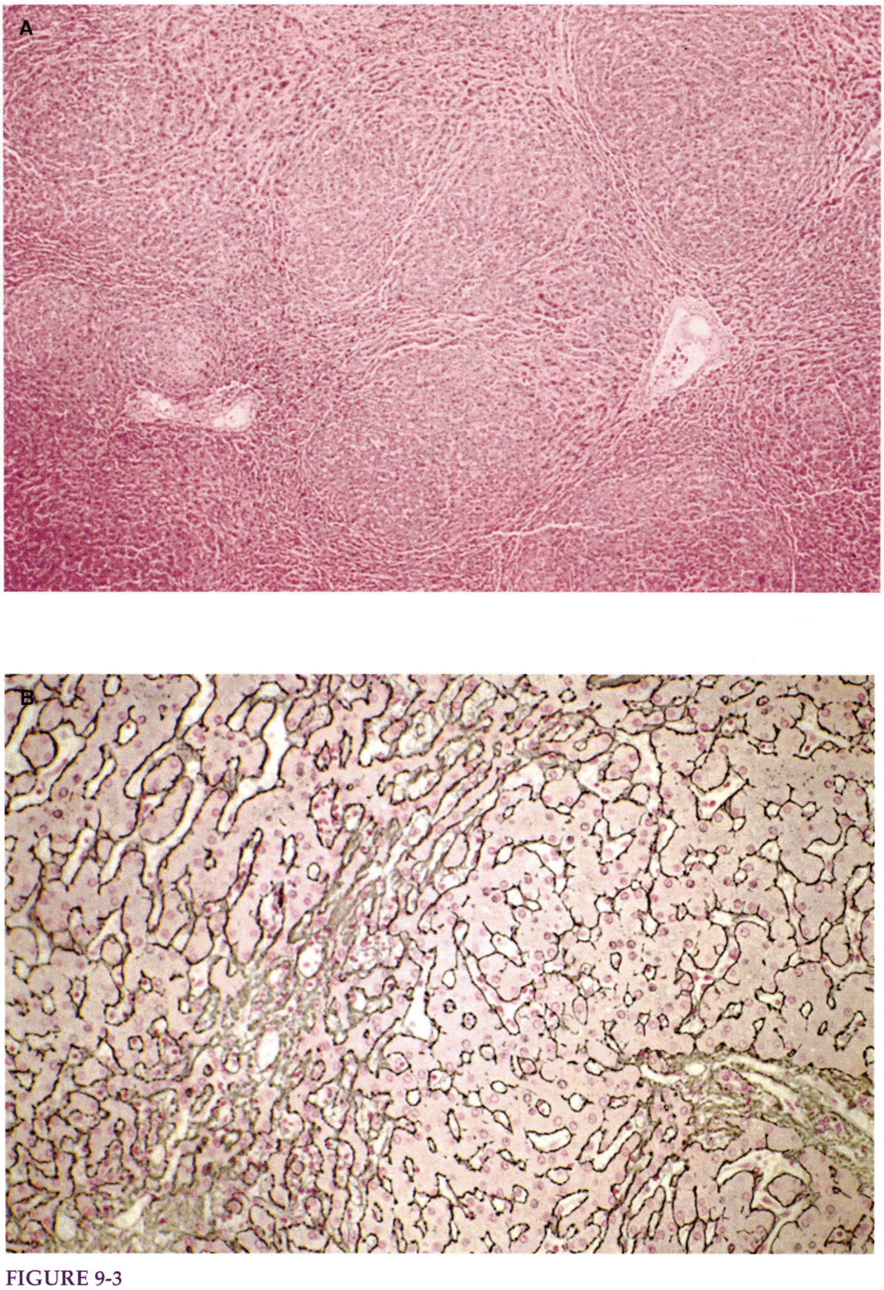

FIGURE 9-3

FIGURE 9-3 (A) NRH. Multiple hepatocellular nodules in a background of mildly atrophic parenchyma (alternating hyperplasia and atrophy pattern). (B) Reticulin stain highlights nodularity.

(*continued*)

Nodular Regenerative Hyperplasia *(continued)*

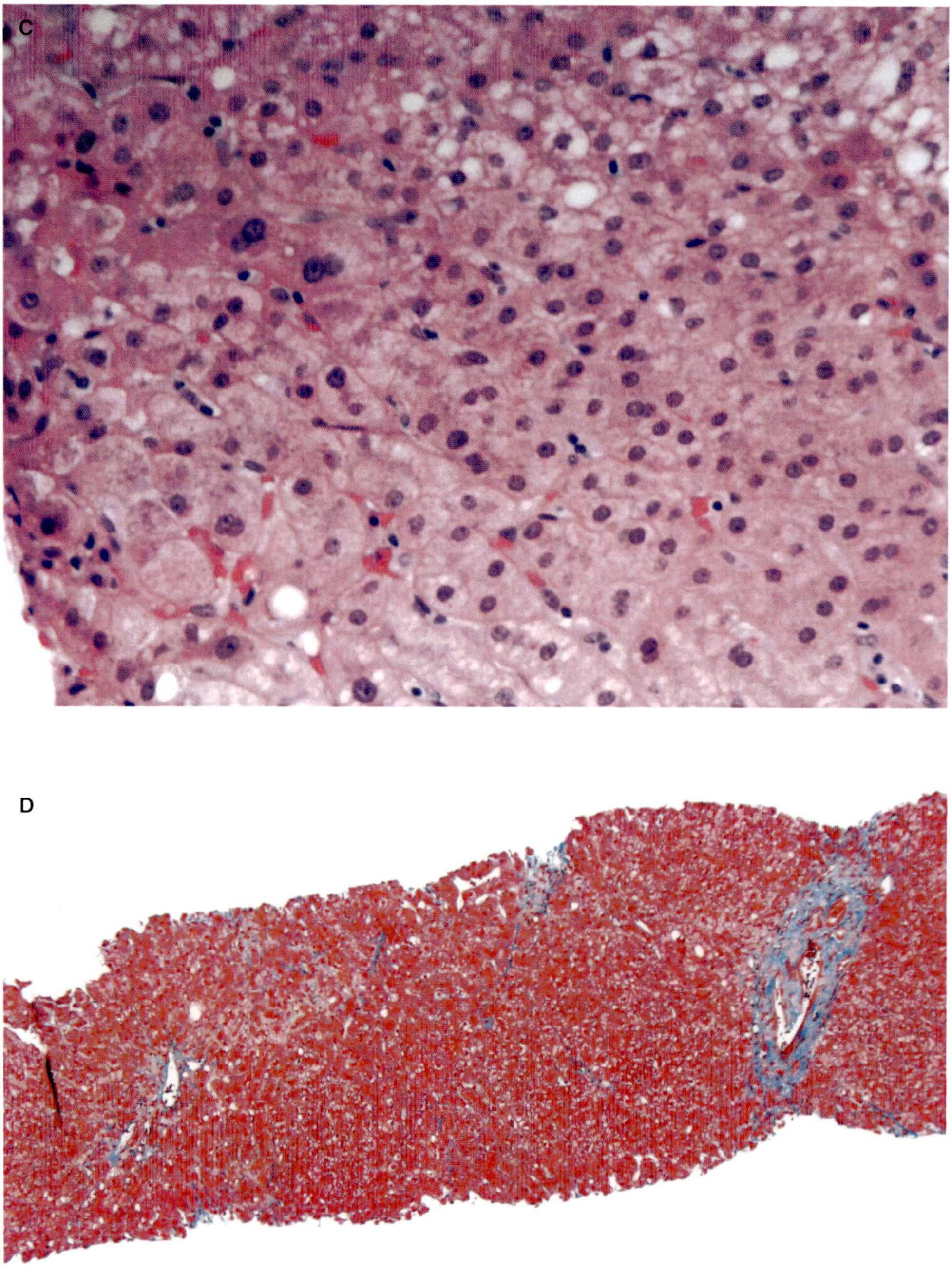

FIGURE 9-3

FIGURE 9-3 (C) Variation in the size of hepatocytes is noted. Areas with smaller cells show increased density of nuclei. (D) Trichrome stain showing lack of fibrosis.

10

Malignant Epithelial Tumors

HEPATOCELLULAR CARCINOMA (HCC)

FIBROLAMELLAR HEPATOCELLULAR CARCINOMA (FLHC)

INTRAHEPATIC CHOLANGIOCARCINOMA (ICC)

COMBINED HEPATOCELLULAR-
CHOLANGIOCARCINOMA (CHCC)

PRIMARY HEPATIC NEUROENDOCRINE TUMOR (PHNET)

METASTATIC CARCINOMA

Hepatocellular Carcinoma (HCC)

DEFINITION

A malignant hepatocellular tumor that usually arises in cirrhotic liver

CLINICAL FEATURES

- Sixth most common malignancy worldwide, with an incidence of about 748,000 new cases diagnosed per year, causing more than 600,000 annual deaths; incidence increasing due to hepatitis C
- Usually occurs in the sixth and seventh decades of life in North America, with lower mean ages at diagnosis in other parts of the world
- Male:female ratio 8:1 in cirrhotic cases, 2–3:1 in noncirrhotic cases
- Can be asymptomatic or present with abdominal pain, weight loss, jaundice, ascites, malaise, and fever
- Elevated alpha-fetoprotein (typically 1,000–100,000 ng/mL)

PATHOLOGIC FEATURES

- Solitary or multiple, most cases with a cirrhotic background (Figure 10-1A)
- Mostly larger than, or exhibiting a color (green if bile-stained, pale if steatotic) and texture different from, the surrounding cirrhotic nodules (Figure 10-1A)
- Microscopically, hepatocellular trabeculli or plates thicker than 3-cell layers; loss of normal reticulin framework (Figure 10-1B)
- Tumor cells mostly retain features of hepatocytes (large polygonal cells with abundant eosinophilic, granular cytoplasm, round central nucleus, and a low to moderate nucleus-to-cytoplasm ratio) (Figures 10-1B, C)
- Immunohistochemically, various patterns seen but mostly positive for HepPar-1, arginase-1, glypican-3, and alpha-fetoprotein; polyclonal CEA and CD10 are expressed in a canalicular pattern (Figure 10-1D)
- Architectural variants: trabecular/sinusoidal, acinar/adenoid/pseudoglandular, solid/compact, and scirrhous
- Cytologic variants: sarcomatoid (abundant spindle cells), pleomorphic (numerous giant cells), and clear cell (numerous clear cells)

DIFFERENTIAL DIAGNOSIS IN A CIRRHOTIC LIVER

- Cirrhotic nodule
- Macroregenerative nodule
- Dysplastic nodule
- Metastasis

DIFFERENTIAL DIAGNOSIS IN A NONCIRRHOTIC LIVER

- Metastasis (pulmonary, pancreatic, colonic, gastric, mammary adenocarcinomas)
- Hepatic adenoma
- Focal nodular hyperplasia
- Cholangiocarcinoma
- Mesenchymal neoplasms

DIFFERENTIAL DIAGNOSIS FOR WELL-DIFFERENTIATED HCC

- Hepatic adenoma

DIFFERENTIAL DIAGNOSIS FOR POORLY DIFFERENTIATED HCC

- Cholangiocarcinoma
- Metastatic adenocarcinoma

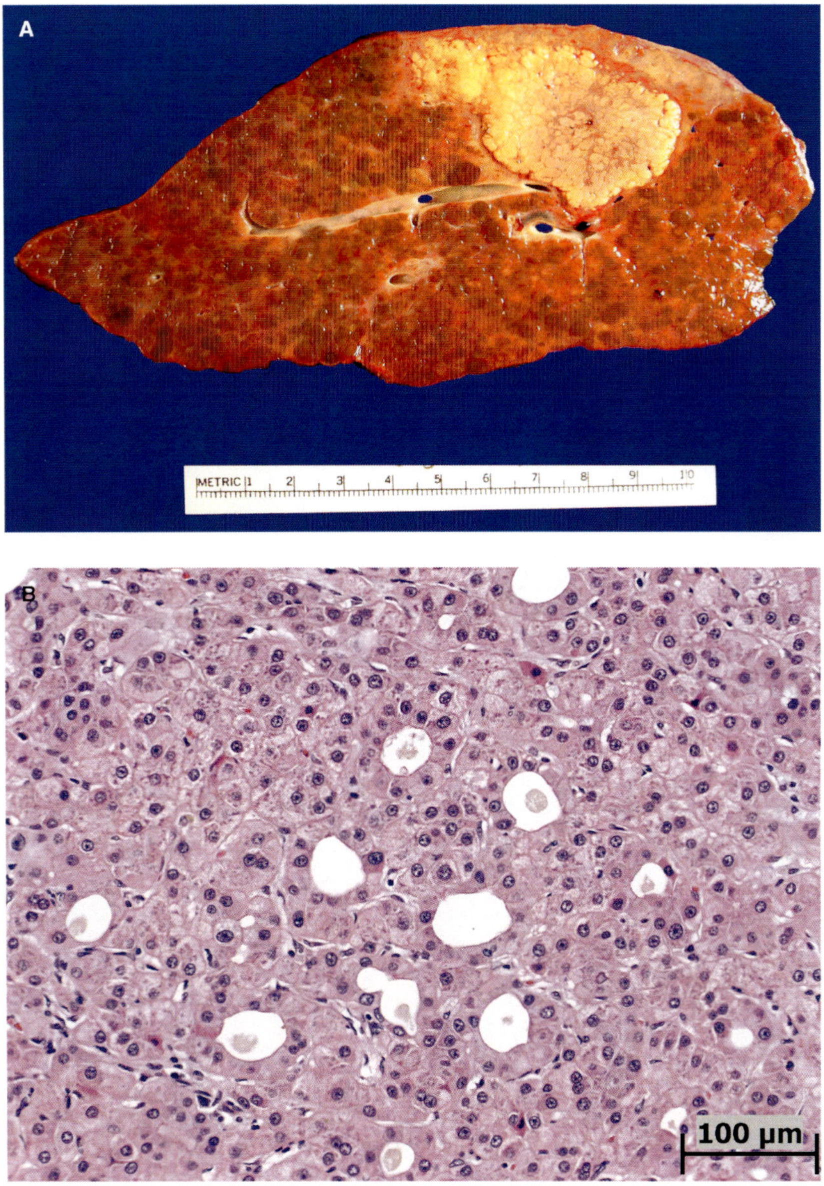

FIGURE 10-1

FIGURE 10-1 (A) HCC in a cirrhotic liver due to hepatitis C. The tumor is necrotic due to treatment. (B) Well-differentiated HCC. Note prominent pseudo-acinar formation. The tumor cells otherwise exhibit typical hepatocytic morphology with low to moderate grade nuclei.

(*continued*)

Hepatocellular Carcinoma (HCC) *(continued)*

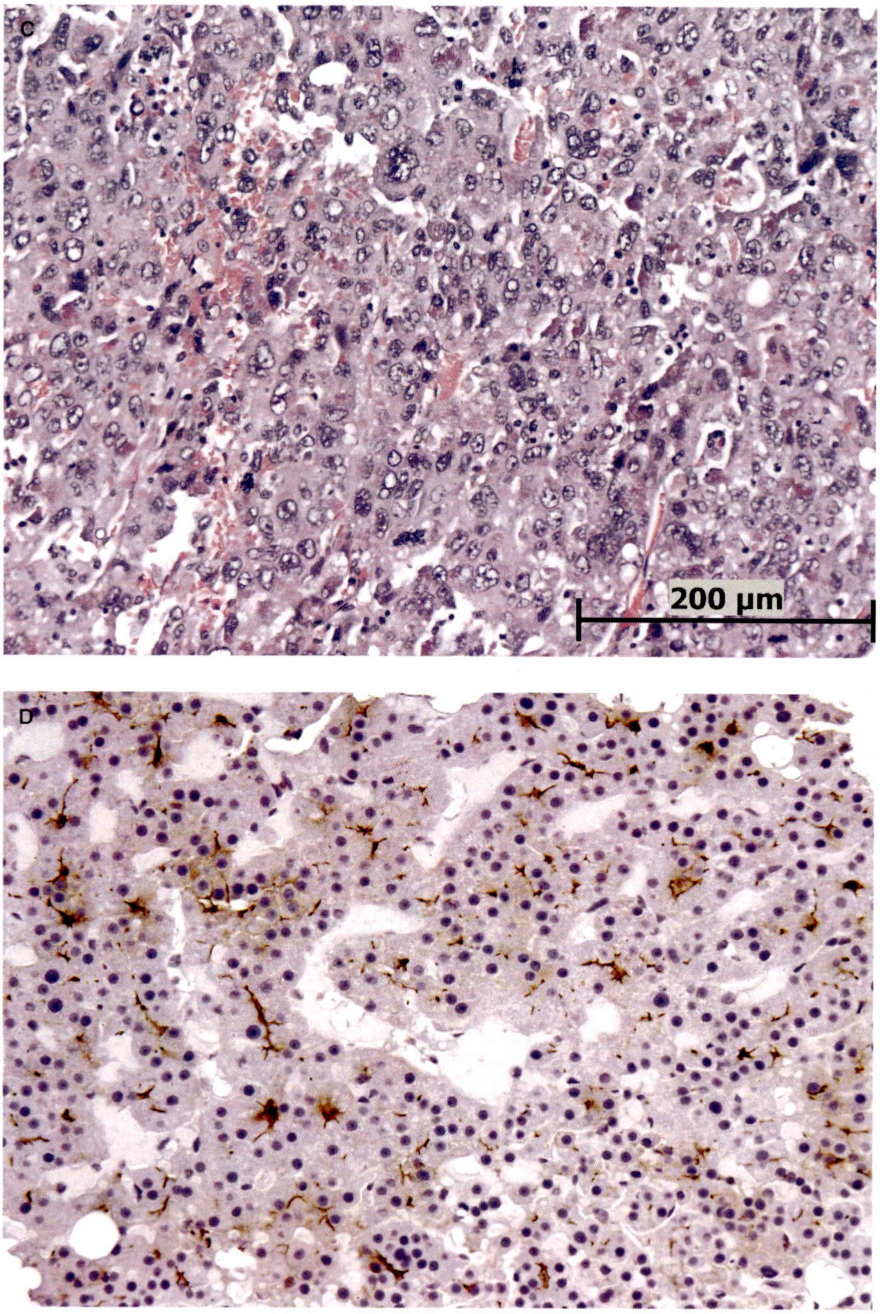

FIGURE 10-1

FIGURE 10-1 (C) Poorly differentiated HCC. Tumor cells with high-grade nuclei irregularly arranged in sheets. (D) Immunostain for CD10 showing the canalicular pattern in a well-differentiated HCC.

Fibrolamellar Hepatocellular Carcinoma (FLHC)

DEFINITION

A special type of hepatocellular carcinoma with a characteristic morphology of parallel fibrous lamella, mostly in young adults and pediatric patients, and not associated with cirrhosis

CLINICAL FEATURES

- Most patients diagnosed before 25 years of age
- Male:female ratio of 1:1
- May present with abdominal pain, large mass, intra-abdominal bleeding, weight loss or jaundice
- Normal serum alpha-fetoprotein level
- Better prognosis than conventional hepatocellular carcinoma (5-year survival rate 50%) in general, due to lack of cirrhosis; similar prognosis when matched stage-for-stage to other cases of HCC without cirrhosis

PATHOLOGIC FEATURES

- Large, usually solitary mass (Figure 10-2A)
- Well-defined lobular pattern, with grossly visible fibrous septa or central scar (Figure 10-2A)
- Tumor cells arranged in cords, nests, or sheets, usually separated or surrounded by lamellar fibrosis (Figures 10-2B, C)
- Deeply eosinophilic, granular, even oncocytic cytoplasm, often containing hyaline globules (alpha-1-antitrypsin), or pale bodies (fibrinogen and albumin) (Figures 10-2B, C, D)
- Normal background (no cirrhosis)
- Immunohistochemically, positive for HepPar-1, CK7, EMA, and may be reactive for neuroendocrine markers

DIFFERENTIAL DIAGNOSIS

- Hepatic adenoma
- Focal nodular hyperplasia
- Hepatocellular carcinoma, scirrhous variant

(*continued*)

Fibrolamellar Hepatocellular Carcinoma (FLHC) *(continued)*

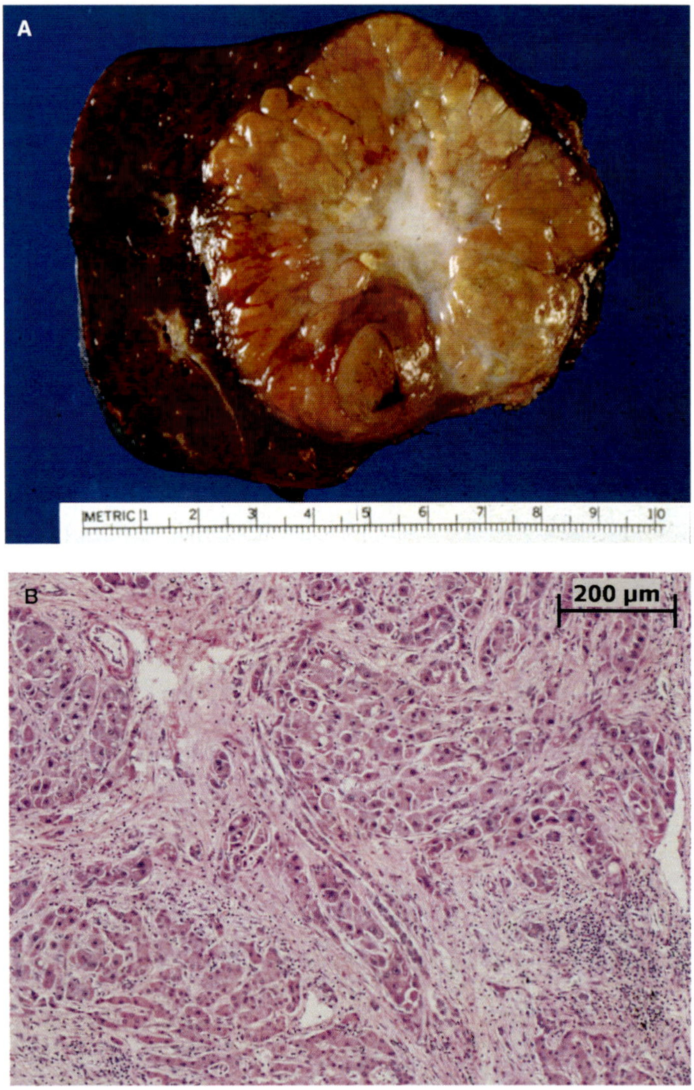

FIGURE 10-2

FIGURE 10-2 (A) Fibrolamellar hepatocellular carcinoma. A well-circumscribed, large, solitary mass with a central scar, in a background of noncirrhotic parenchyma. (B) Fibrous septa traverse the tumor, separating cords and nests of tumor cells.

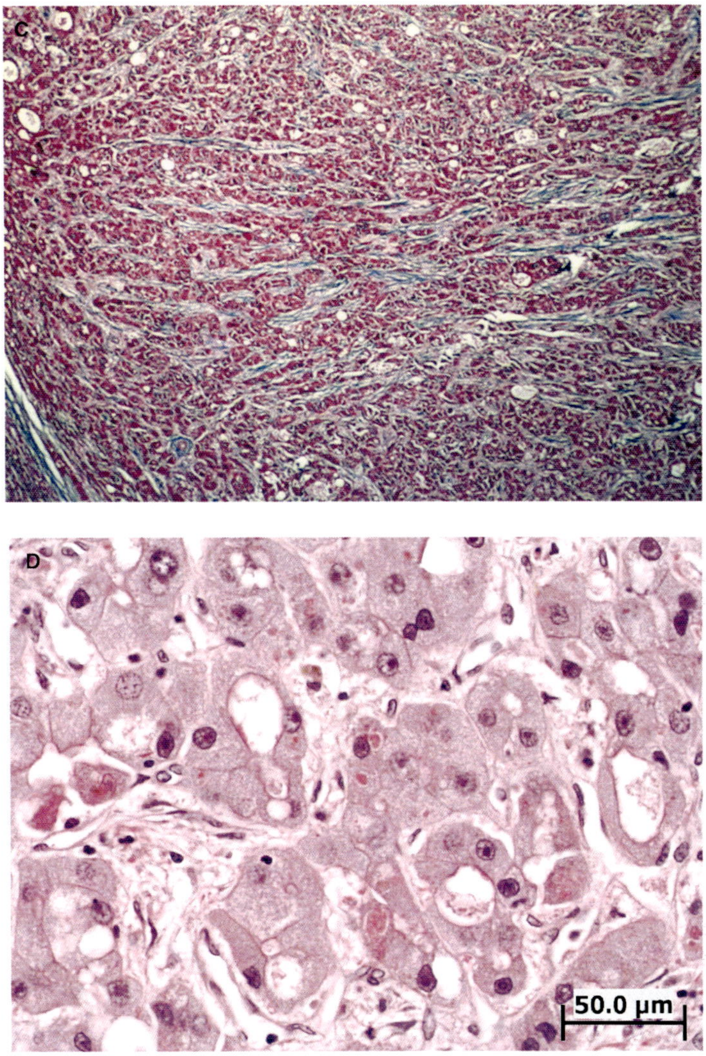

FIGURE 10-2

FIGURE 10-2 (C) Trichrome stain highlights the fibrous (collagenous) strands. (D) Tumor cells with abundant eosinophilic oncocytic cytoplasm, occasionally containing cytoplasmic globules. Pseudoacinar formation is also present.

Intrahepatic Cholangiocarcinoma (ICC)

DEFINITION

Adenocarcinoma arising from the intrahepatic bile ducts

CLINICAL FEATURES

- Constitutes 5–15% of primary hepatic malignancies
- Male:female ratio of 1:1; mostly 60 years of age
- Most cases have no history of cirrhosis

PATHOLOGIC FEATURES

- Mostly poorly differentiated adenocarcinoma with infiltrative growth (Figures 10-3A, B)
- Tumor cells spread between hepatocellular plates and along ducts and nerves; lymphatic invasion common (Figures 10-3C, B)
- Marked desmoplastic reaction and abundant fibrous stroma (Figures 10-3D, B)
- Background liver parenchyma usually noncirrhotic
- Immunohistochemically positive for CK7, negative for CK20 and CDX2, and negative for other hepatocytic markers

DIFFERENTIAL DIAGNOSIS

- Metastatic extrahepatic pancreatobiliary carcinoma
- Metastatic adenocarcinoma of other origins
- Poorly differentiated hepatocellular carcinoma
- Bile duct hamartoma
- Combined hepatocellular-cholangiocarcinoma

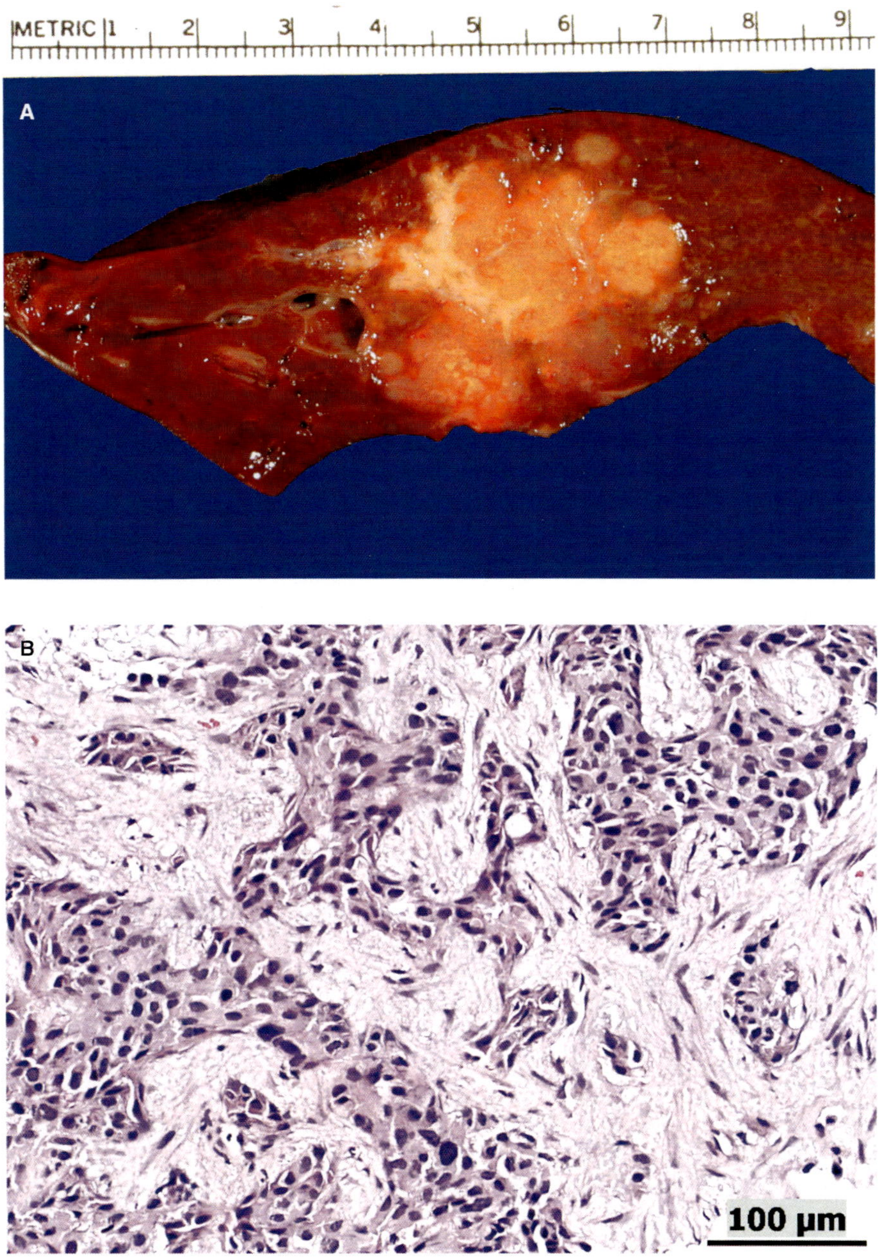

FIGURE 10-3

FIGURE 10-3 (A) Cholangiocarcinoma from a 78-year-old male. Irregular mass with an infiltrative edge and small satellite lesions, in a noncirrhotic liver. (B) Poorly differentiated cholangiocarcinoma.

(*continued*)

Intrahepatic Cholangiocarcinoma (ICC) *(continued)*

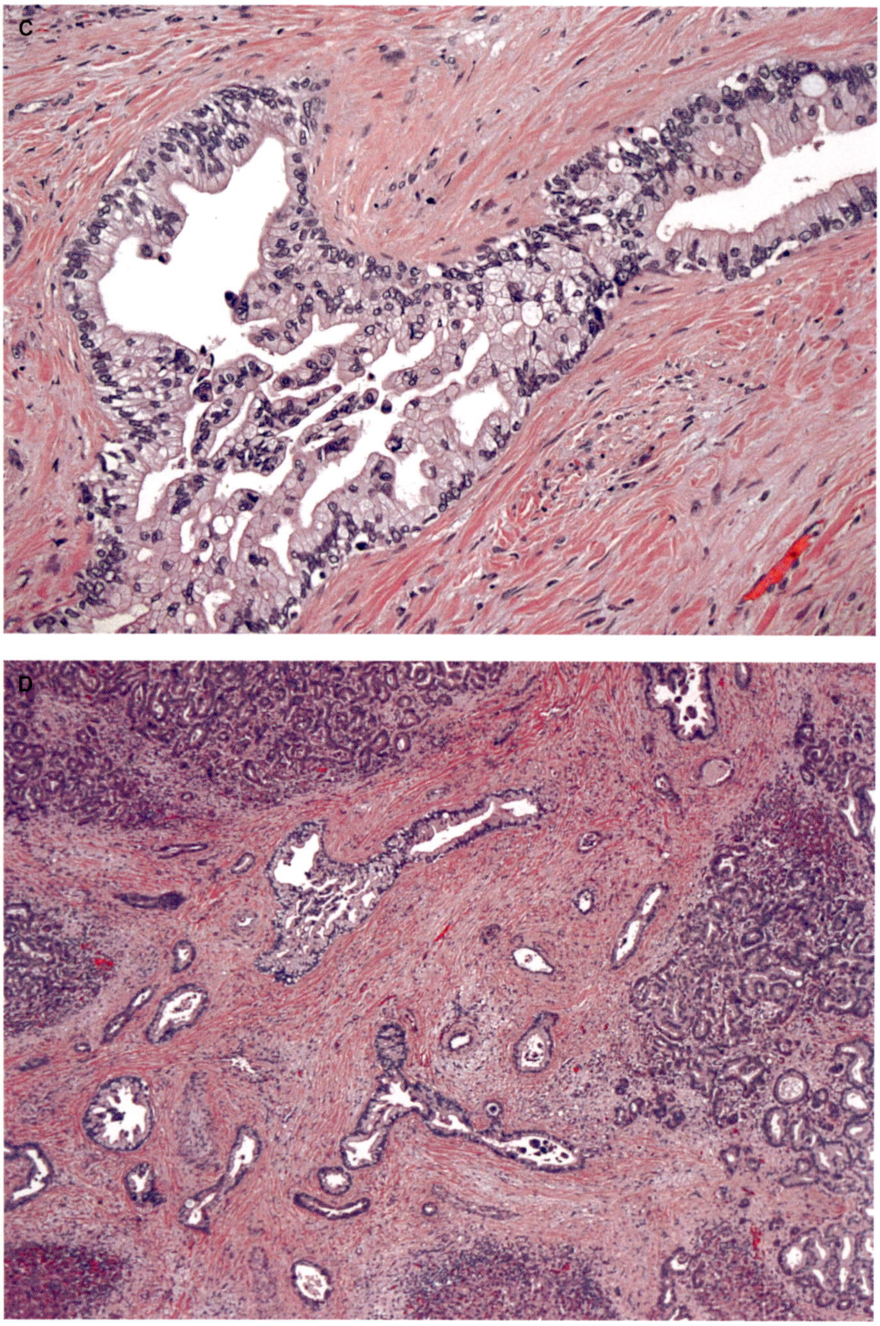

FIGURE 10-3

FIGURE 10-3 (C) Higher power view of the intraductal component. (D) The tumor consists of nodules of well-formed small glands in dense fibrotic stroma; intraductal papillary neoplasia with high-grade dysplasia is evident.

Combined Hepatocellular-Cholangiocarcinoma (CHCC)

DEFINITION

A tumor with components of both HCC and CC; less than 5% of primary liver malignancies

CLINICAL FEATURES

- Similar to that of HCC

PATHOLOGIC FEATURES

- Typical features of HCC (trabeculli and/or acinar formation, bile production or canaliculi) (Figures 10-4A, B)
- Typical features of CC (biliary epithelial phenotype with desmoplastic stroma) (Figures 10-4A, C)
- Immunostains demonstrating the above phenotypes corresponding to either element (CEA-p, HepPar-1, arginase, CD10, for the HCC component; CK19, MOC31 for the CC component) (Figure 10-4D)

DIFFERENTIAL DIAGNOSIS

- Conventional HCC
- Intrahepatic cholangiocarcinoma

(*continued*)

Combined Hepatocellular-Cholangiocarcinoma (CHCC) *(continued)*

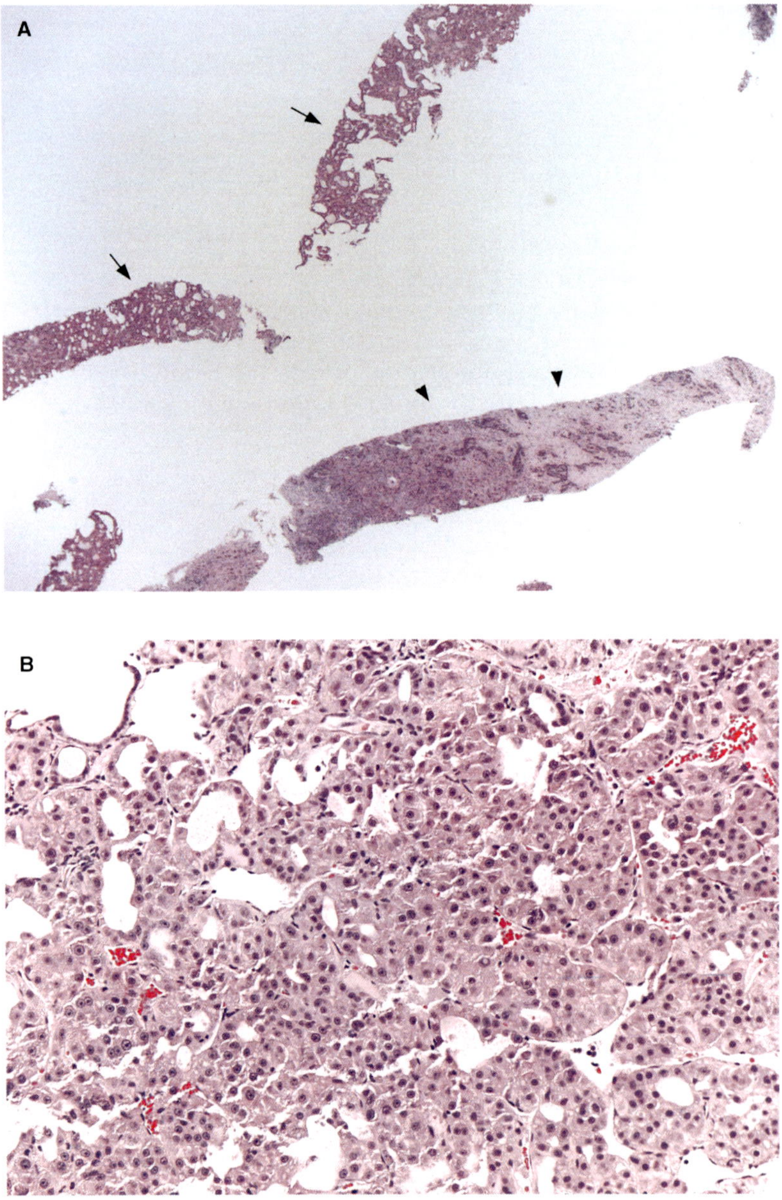

FIGURE 10-4

FIGURE 10-4 (A) Mixed hepatocellular-cholangiocarcinoma. Fragments of needle biopsies containing typical well-differentiated HCC (arrows) and poorly differentiated carcinoma (arrowheads). (B) High power view of HCC.

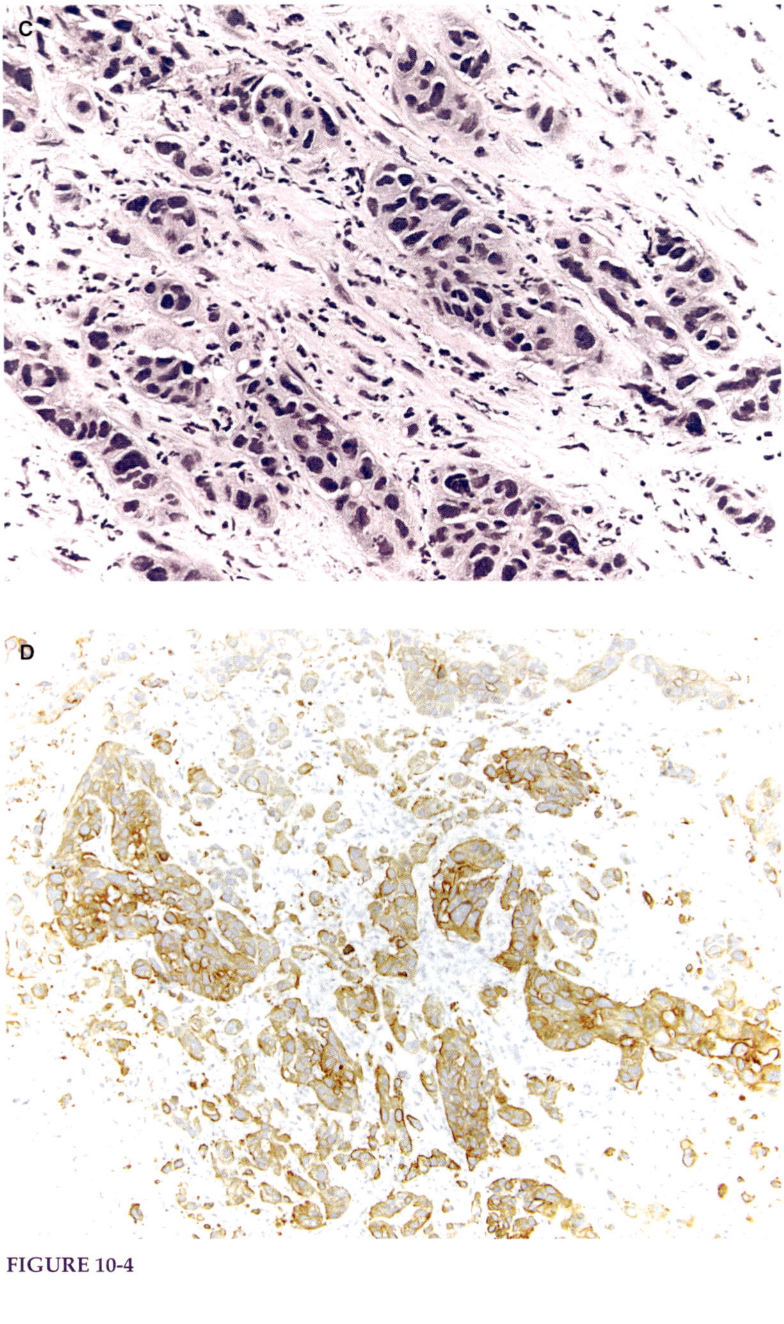

FIGURE 10-4

FIGURE 10-4 (C) High power view of the poorly differentiated carcinoma. (D) Immunostain for CK19 is positive in the cholangiocarcinoma component (not shown: HepPar-1 and arginase-1 negative; MOC-31 positive).

Primary Hepatic Neuroendocrine Tumor (PHNET)

DEFINITION

Rare well-differentiated neuroendocrine tumor (carcinoid tumor) occurring in the liver, with metastasis ruled out by extensive clinical work up

CLINICAL FEATURES

- Asymptomatic or present with an abdominal mass, slow growing
- Indolent clinical course and radiographic features may lead to clinical misdiagnosis as a hemangioma

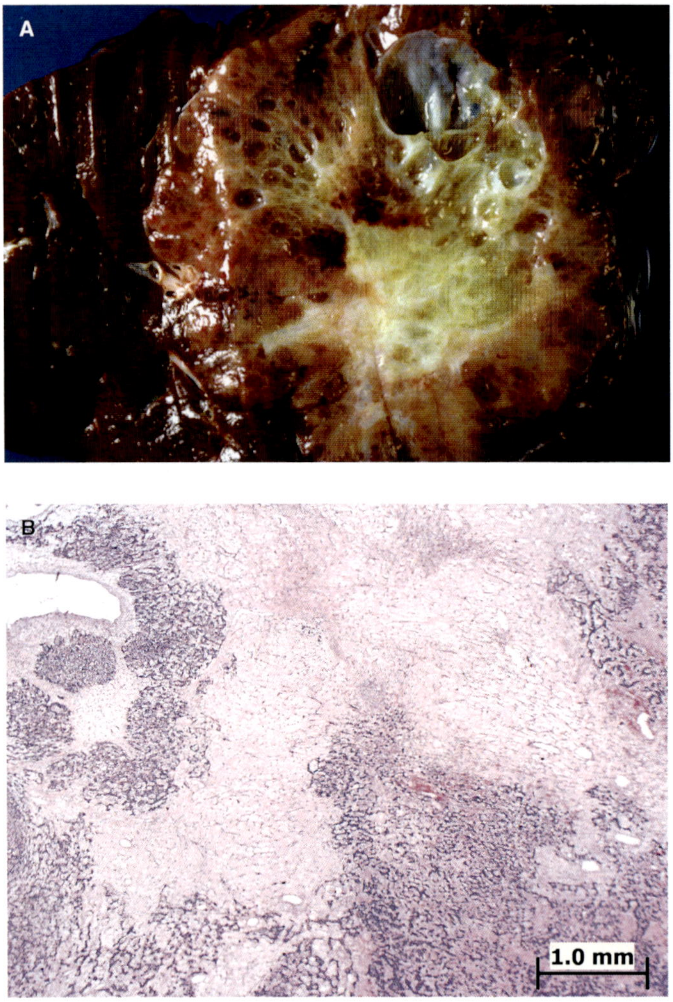

FIGURE 10-5

FIGURE 10-5 (A) Primary hepatic neuroendocrine tumor. A solitary mass in a noncirrhotic liver. The cut surface demonstrates central degeneration, with prominent macro- and microcystic changes. (B) Extensive intratumoral edematous degeneration, mixed with thin anastomosing cords of tumor cells.

PATHOLOGIC FEATURES

- Solitary large mass, well-circumscribed (Figure 10-5A)
- Large areas of degenerative change due to slow growth and large size, often with cystic or microcystic cut surface (Figure 10-5A)
- Corresponding microscopic changes: degeneration, cyst formation (including blood-filled microcysts), and focal pseudoglandular formation (Figure 10-5B)
- Tumor cells otherwise indistinguishable from other carcinoid tumors (Figures 10-5C, D)

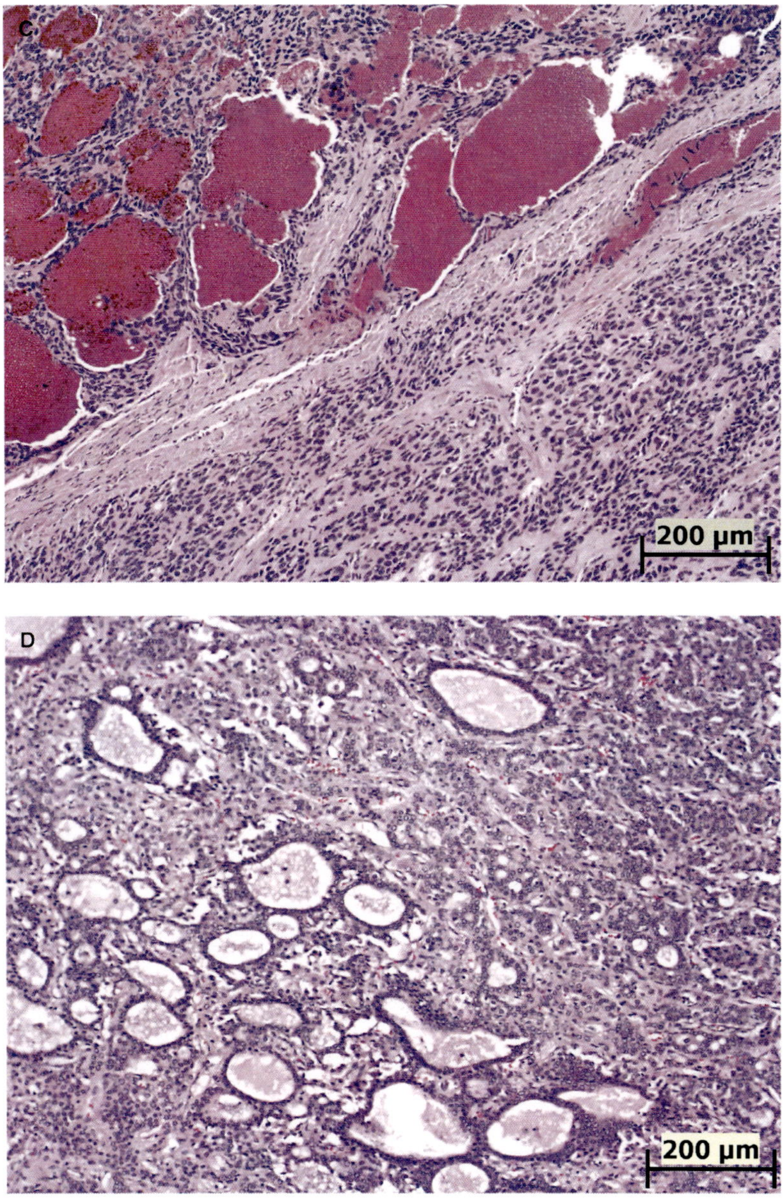

FIGURE 10-5

FIGURE 10-5 (C) Blood-filled microcysts. (D) Pseudoglandular formation is focally prominent.

Metastatic Carcinoma

DEFINITION

Several commonly encountered metastatic carcinomas are discussed in this section.

CLINICAL FEATURES

- Higher prevalence than primary malignancies in Western countries; the difference is less remarkable in Asia
- Known history of a previously diagnosed tumor most helpful in the diagnosis and determining the origin of a metastasis
- Further clinical work-up including comprehensive imaging studies required if the metastasis is the initial diagnosis (lack of a previously diagnosed tumor)

PATHOLOGIC FEATURES

- Some carcinomas have characteristic microscopic features (breast, pancreaticobiliary, ovary, neuroendocrine, sarcoma, etc.) (Figures 10-6A–D).
- Metastasis from renal cell carcinoma (Figure 10-6B), adrenal cortical carcinoma, and melanoma mimic HCC on H&E sections.
- Metastasis from extrahepatic biliary tree or pancreas indistinguishable from primary intrahepatic cholangiocarcinoma histologically.
- Most carcinoid tumors are metastases (Figure 10-6D), except for very rare cases.
- Various combinations of immunostains can help determine the origin or phenotype of tumor cells (colorectal adenocarcinoma is positive for CK20 and CDX2 but negative for CK7; hormone receptor status for breast carcinoma; TTF-1 for lung cancer, etc.).

DIFFERENTIAL DIAGNOSIS

- Intrahepatic cholangiocarcinoma
- Hepatocellular carcinoma
- Bile duct hamartoma

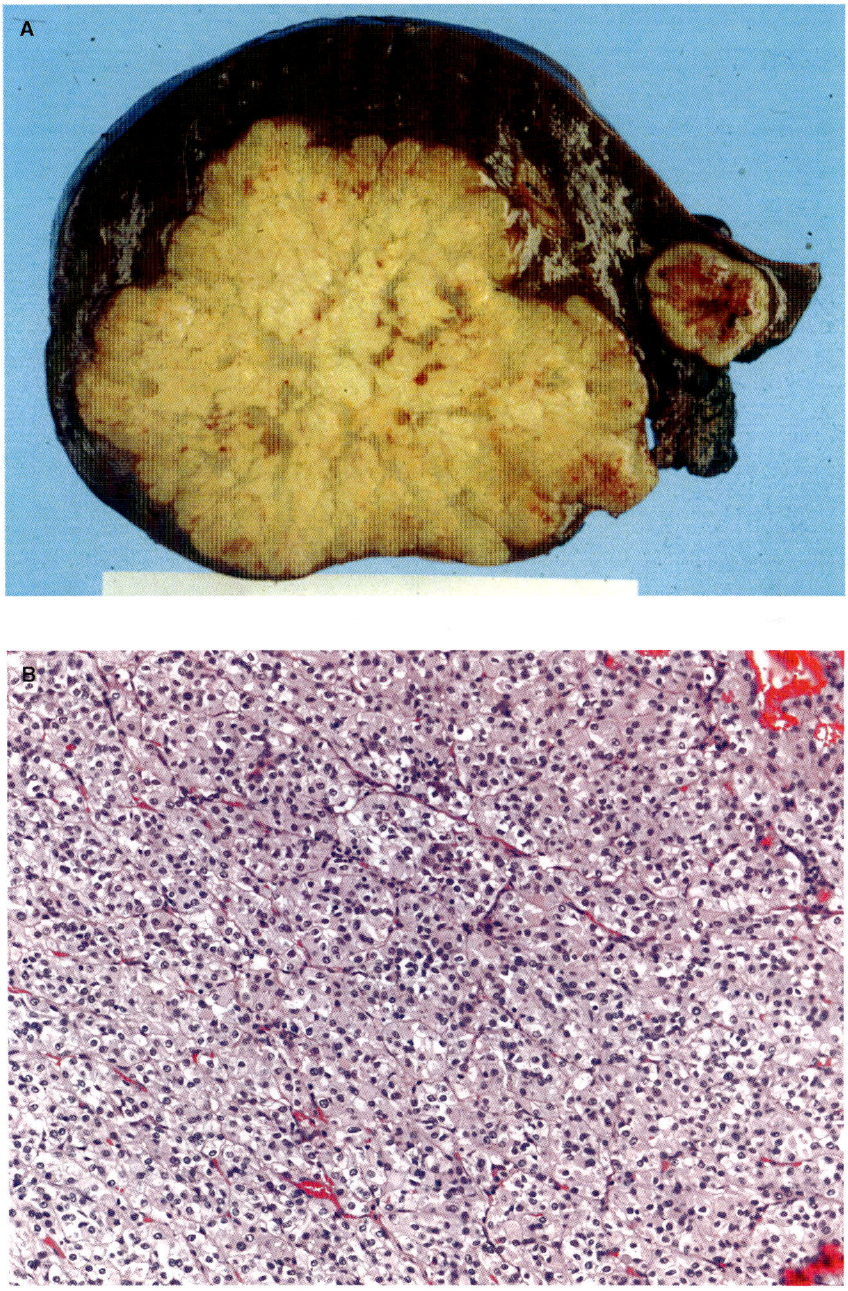

FIGURE 10-6

FIGURE 10-6 (A) Metastatic colonic adenocarcinoma: well-demarcated mass with a satellite lesion, in a background of normal parenchyma. (B) Metastatic renal cell carcinoma. The tumor consists of thick trabecula or nests of large cells with abundant somewhat granular eosinophilic cytoplasms, mimicking HCC.

(*continued*)

Metastatic Carcinoma *(continued)*

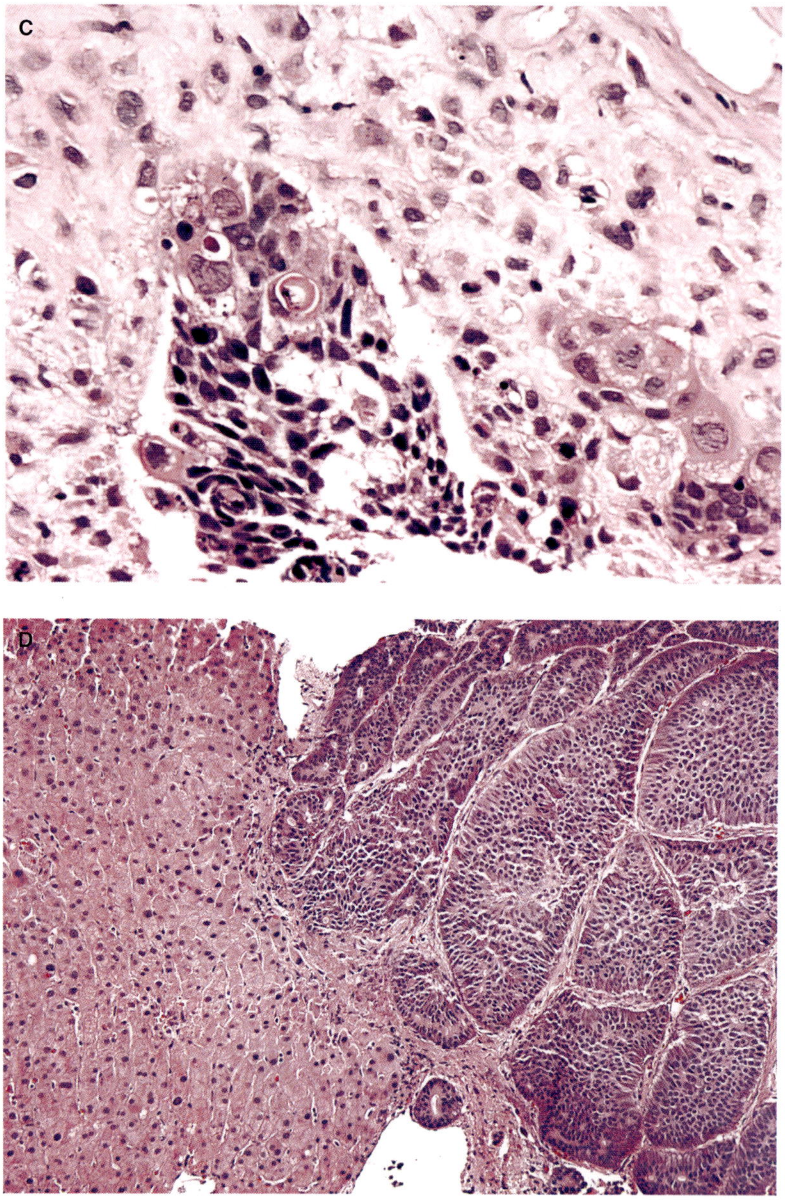

FIGURE 10-6

FIGURE 10-6 (C) An unusual metastatic carcinoma from a prostate primary, with focal squamous cell differentiation. Review of the original prostatectomy specimen revealed focal squamous differentiation (case courtesy of Dr. Xiuli Liu). (D) Metastatic small bowel carcinoid tumor.

Vascular Tumors

11

HEMANGIOMA

EPITHELIOID HEMANGIOENDOTHELIOMA

INFANTILE HEMANGIOENDOTHELIOMA

ANGIOSARCOMA

Hemangioma

DEFINITION

A benign vascular tumor, hemangioma is likely the most common benign liver tumor. Most cases exhibit the morphology of a cavernous hemangioma, although partial or complete sclerosis may occur in others, giving rise to sclerosing hemangiomas or solitary fibrous nodules.

CLINICAL FEATURES

- No age or gender predilections
- Many cases asymptomatic and incidentally discovered
- Large lesions may cause symptoms: abdominal pain or discomfort, palpable mass, bleeding from ruptured giant tumors

PATHOLOGIC FEATURES

- Usually solitary, 5 cm or smaller
- Well-delineated, mostly subcapsular (Figure 11-1A)
- Histologically cavernous vascular spaces, with flat endothelial cells, fibrous stroma (Figures 11-1B and C)
- Sclerotic tumors common, with scattered irregular and small endothelium-lined channels or cords (Figure 11-1D)

DIFFERENTIAL DIAGNOSIS

- Peliosis
- Angiosarcoma
- Sclerotic bile duct hamartoma

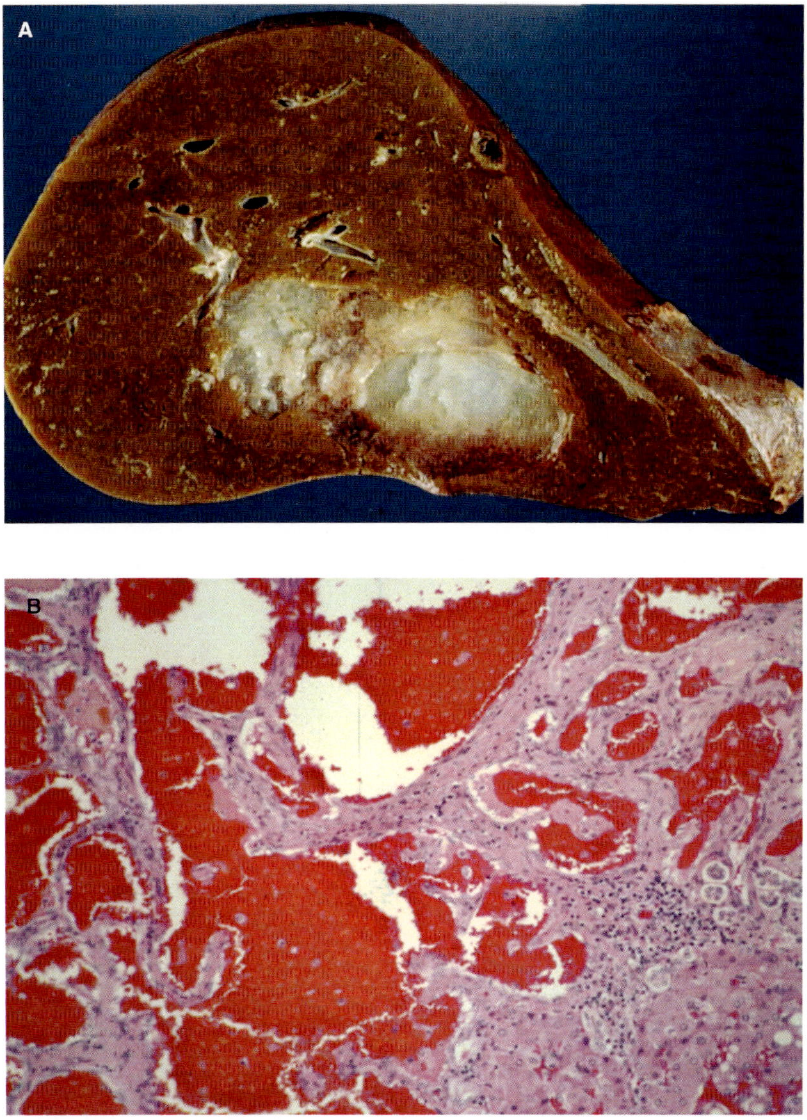

FIGURE 11-1

FIGURE 11-1 (A) Gross photo of a cavernous hemangioma within a background of normal liver parenchyma. (B) Cavernous hemangioma with large, blood-filled, anastomosing vascular channels with prominent fibrous septa.

(*continued*)

Hemangioma *(continued)*

C

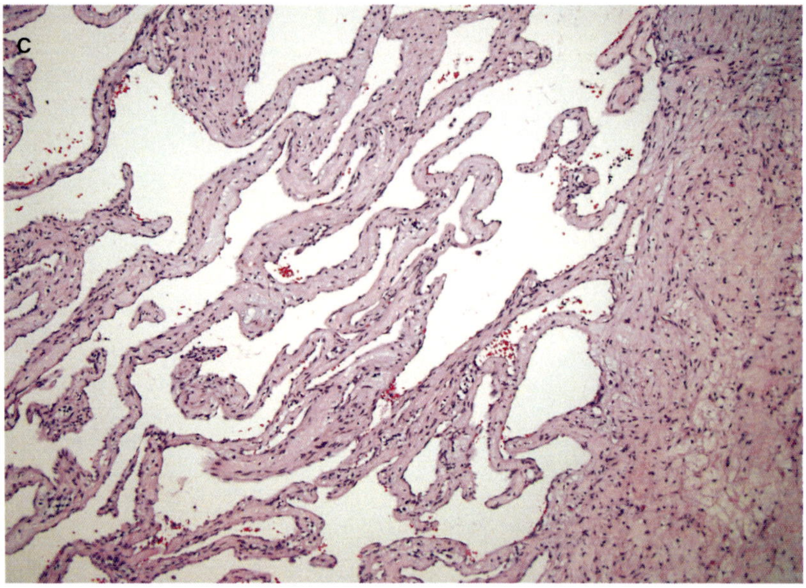

D

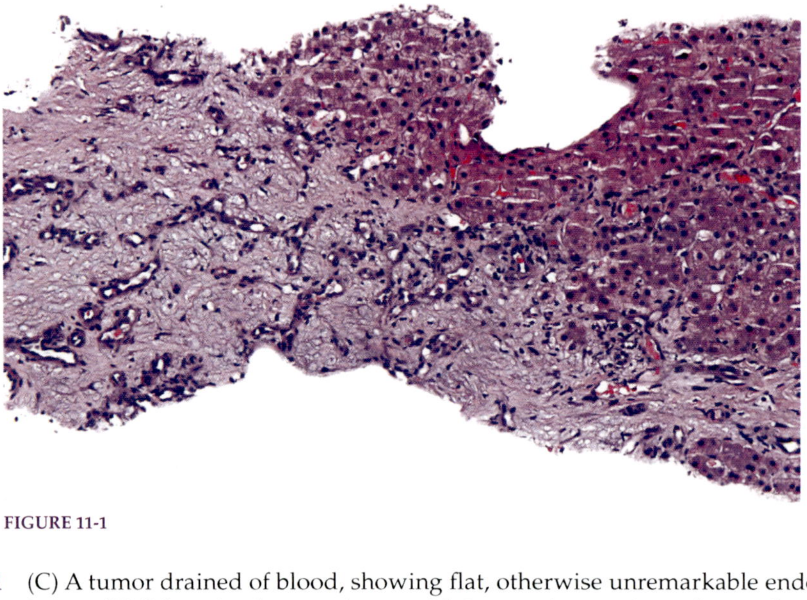

FIGURE 11-1

FIGURE 11-1 (C) A tumor drained of blood, showing flat, otherwise unremarkable endothelial lining. (D) Sclerosing hemangioma, with inconspicuous, irregular cords of benign endothelial cells. Occasionally immunohistochemical stains may be applied to confirm the endothelial nature (versus the epithelial cells of a bile duct hamartoma).

Epithelioid Hemangioendothelioma

DEFINITION

A rare, low-grade malignant vascular tumor of adults, hepatic epithelioid hemangioendothelioma (EHE) consists of dense fibrous stroma and a scattered epithelioid component. Similar counterparts are seen in lung and soft tissue.

CLINICAL FEATURES

- Average age 50 years; male-to-female ratio 1:2
- Presentation: abdominal pain
- Radiologically, multiple nodular lesions
- Elevated serum alkaline phosphatase level in some cases
- Patients may die of progressive liver failure or metastatic disease
- Liver transplantation is treatment of choice

PATHOLOGIC FEATURES

- Multinodular in majority of cases
- Infiltrative growth (ill-defined border) (Figure 11-2A)
- Dense hyalinized fibrous tissue at center of a lesion, may have calcification; abundant stromal matrix with myxoid or cartilaginous appearance (Figures 11-2B, C)
- Scattered small clusters of tumor cells, with intracellular lumens or small vascular spaces (Figure 11-2C)
- Some cases have tufting or papillary epithelioid growth in thin-walled vascular spaces (Figure 11-2C)
- Immunostains positive for CD31, CD34, factor VIII-related antigen; rarely cytokeratin positive (Figure 11-2D)

DIFFERENTIAL DIAGNOSIS

- Metastatic carcinoma (multiple nodules grossly)
- Sclerosing cholangiocarcinoma
- Angiosarcoma

(*continued*)

Epithelioid Hemangioendothelioma *(continued)*

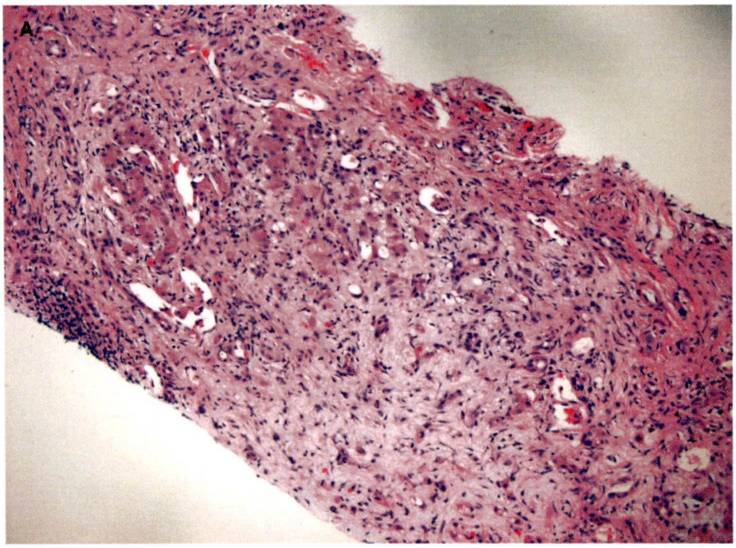

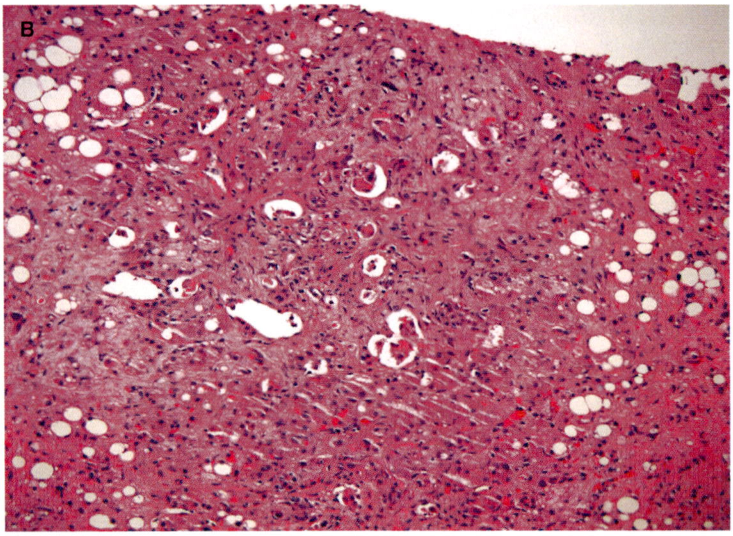

FIGURE 11-2

FIGURE 11-2 (A) EHE with dense fibrous and myxoid stromal areas. Infiltrating the stroma are round single cells with pleomorphic, hyperchromatic nuclei, and scattered vascular channels. Entrapped hepatocytes are also present. (B) Higher magnification of Figure 11-2A, with endothelial cell "tufting" into small vascular spaces.

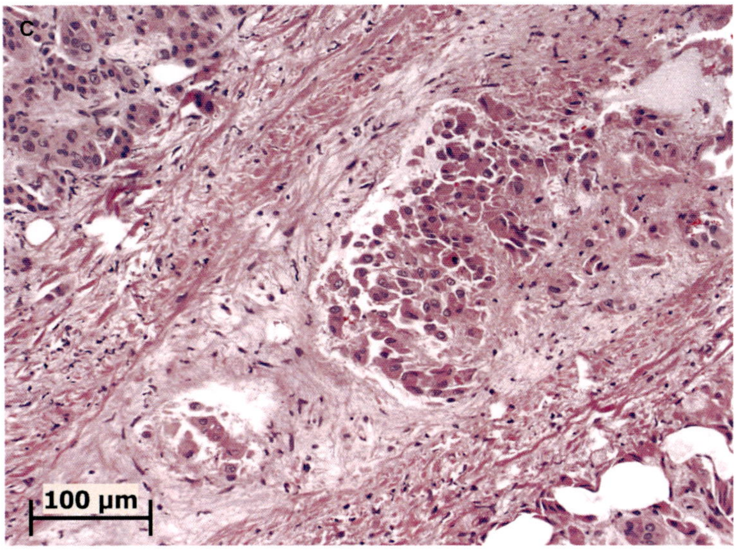

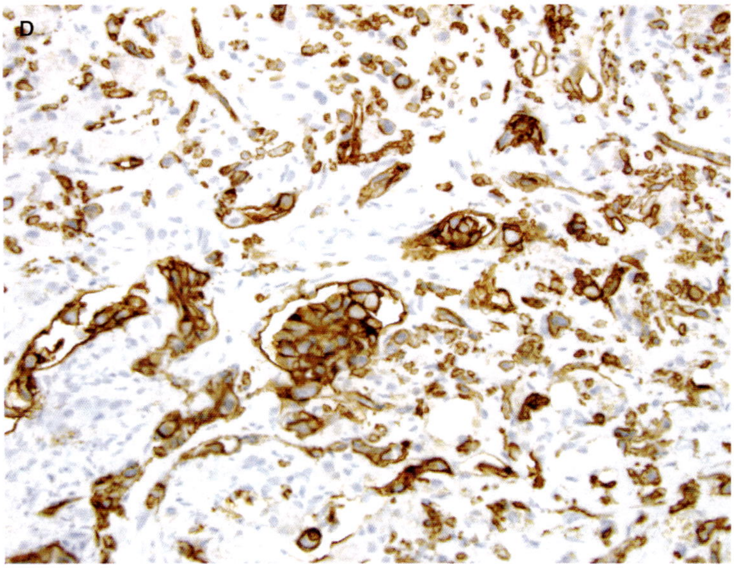

FIGURE 11-2

FIGURE 11-2 (C) EHE. Clusters of large endothelial cells with abundant eosinophilic cytoplasm in vascular spaces. (D) Immunohistochemically, the tumor cells express CD31 (not shown) and CD34.

Infantile Hemangioendothelioma

DEFINITION

A histologically benign vascular tumor, similar to capillary hemangiomas of infancy of the skin and mucosa, which can regress with maturation. However, the tumor can be clinically fatal in some patients due to rupture with hemorrhage, congestive heart failure, or liver failure. This is the second most common liver tumor in children 3 years and under (after hepatoblastoma).

CLINICAL FEATURES

- About 90% of cases diagnosed before 6 months of age, 33% in the first month
- Male-to-female ratio 1:2
- Hepatomegaly or abdominal mass
- Some patients have associated skin hemangiomas
- About 10% of patients have hemangiomas of other organs or other congenital anomalies
- Some patients have high output congestive heart failure

PATHOLOGIC FEATURES

- Single or multicentric, making surgical resection difficult
- Poorly circumscribed, red, brown, or white cut surface, with solid and cystic areas
- Some with central scaring/fibrosis and peripheral vasculature
- Microscopically, small irregular vascular channels, mimicking capillaries, lined by plump endothelial cells; solid areas (Figures 11-3A, B)
- Scant fibrous stroma; entrapped bile ducts or liver parenchyma may be seen at the edges; extramedullary hematopoiesis (Figure 11-3C)
- Central scarring, zones of dystrophic calcification, and hemorrhage are signs of regression
- Occasionally, focal micro-thrombosis (Figure 11-3D)
- Immunomarkers: factor VIII-related antigen, CD31, and CD34

DIFFERENTIAL DIAGNOSIS

- Infantile angiosarcoma
- Congenital vascular malformation

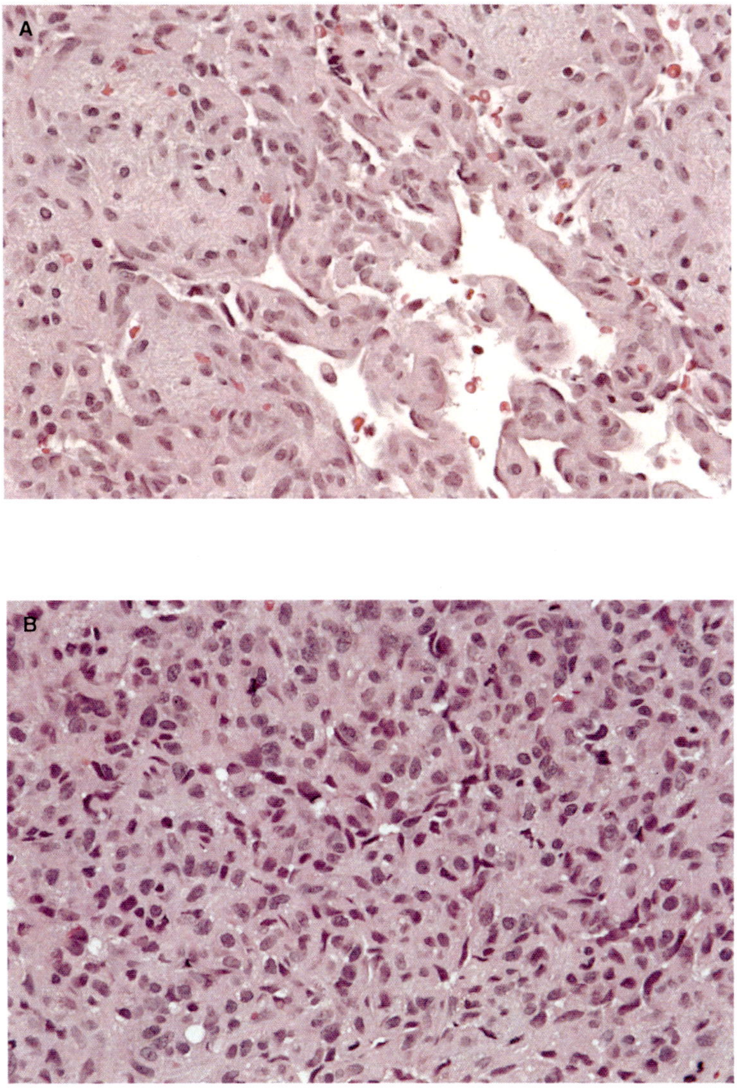

FIGURE 11-3

FIGURE 11-3 (A) Infantile hemangioendothelioma, with small capillary-like vascular channels. (B) Focal solid area, consisting of almost entirely plump endothelial cells.

(continued)

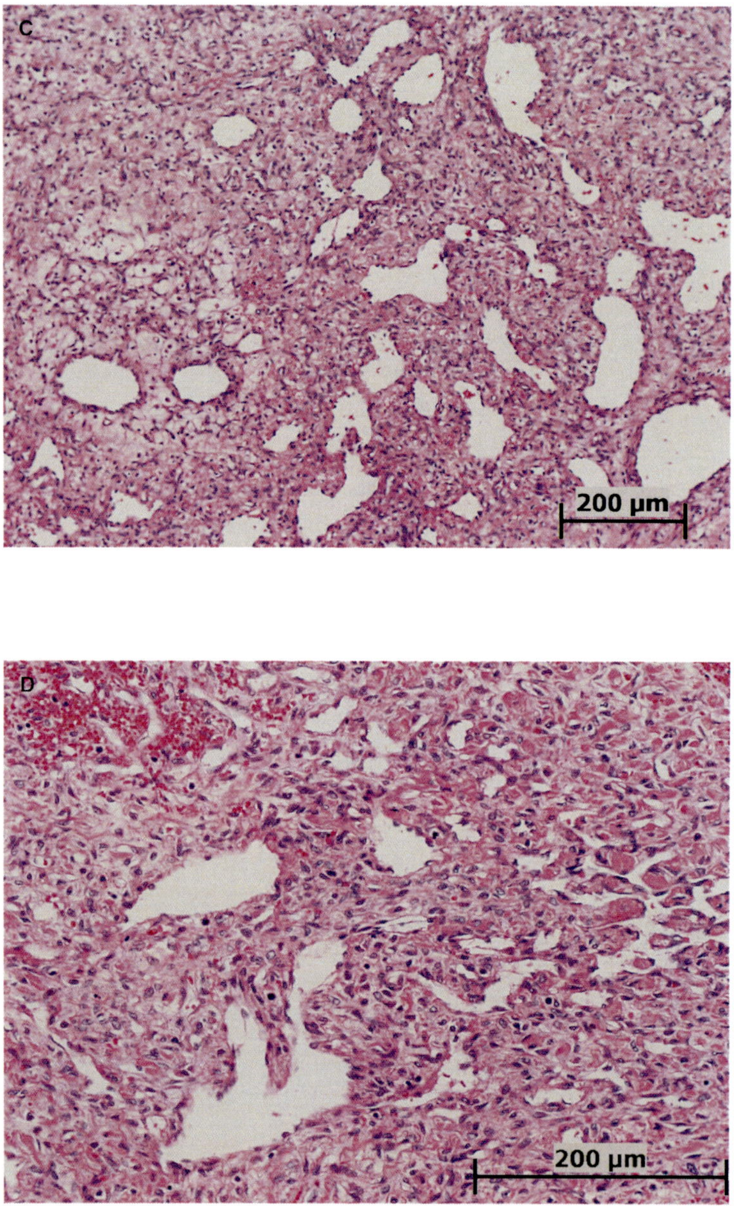

FIGURE 11-3

FIGURE 11-3 (C) Scant fibrous stroma and focal myxoid degeneration (lower right corner). (D) Focal thrombosis at tip of small papillary vessels (middle of the right edge).

Angiosarcoma

DEFINITION

A rare high-grade malignant vascular tumor that is the most common primary sarcoma of the liver. There is a significant association with environmental carcinogens: vinyl chloride monomer, Thorotrast, arsenic, and anabolic steroids in a small proportion of cases.

CLINICAL FEATURES

- Older individuals, peaking in sixth to seventh decade; male-to-female ratio 3:1
- Abdominal pain, abdominal enlargement
- Weight loss, weakness, fatigue, ascites, jaundice
- Abnormal liver enzyme levels
- Thrombocytopenia
- Common outcomes: intra-abdominal or gastrointestinal bleeding
- Most patients die of hepatic failure in 6 months to 1 year of diagnosis

PATHOLOGIC FEATURES

- Hepatomegaly
- Usually multicentric
- Cut surface: multiple nodules with red or brown color, hemorrhagic; solid and cystic areas
- Microscopic: dilated hepatic sinusoids to cavernous vascular channels lined by highly atypical hypertrophic endothelial cells with hyperchromatic nuclei (Figures 11-4A, B)
- Atrophy of hepatocytes
- Solid areas may resemble EHE (Figure 11-4C)
- IHC: factor VIII, CD31, CD34 (Figure 11-4D)

DIFFERENTIAL DIAGNOSIS

- EHE
- Poorly differentiated carcinoma
- Infantile hemangioendothelioma
- Fibrosarcoma
- Inflammatory pseudotumor

(continued)

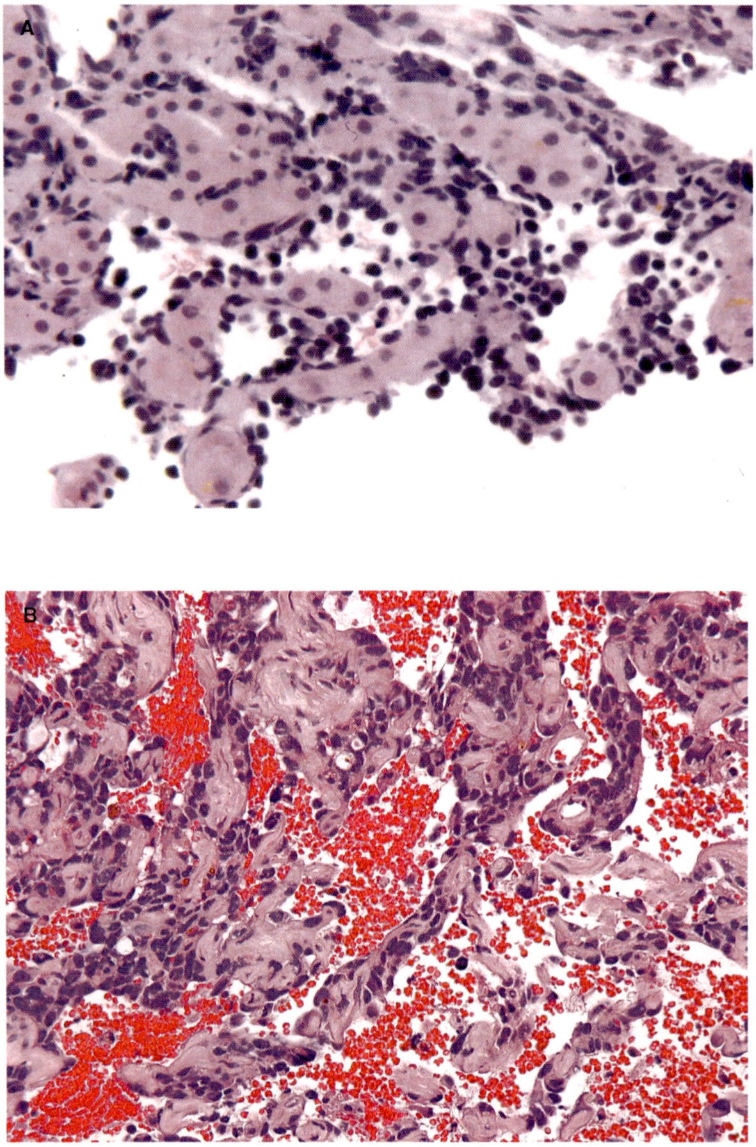

FIGURE 11-4

FIGURE 11-4 (A) Angiosarcoma in a sinusoidal pattern. Note the prominent atypical endothelial cells lining cords of slightly atrophic hepatocytes. (B) Angiosarcoma with cavernous pattern. Note the fibrous septae without hepatocytes.

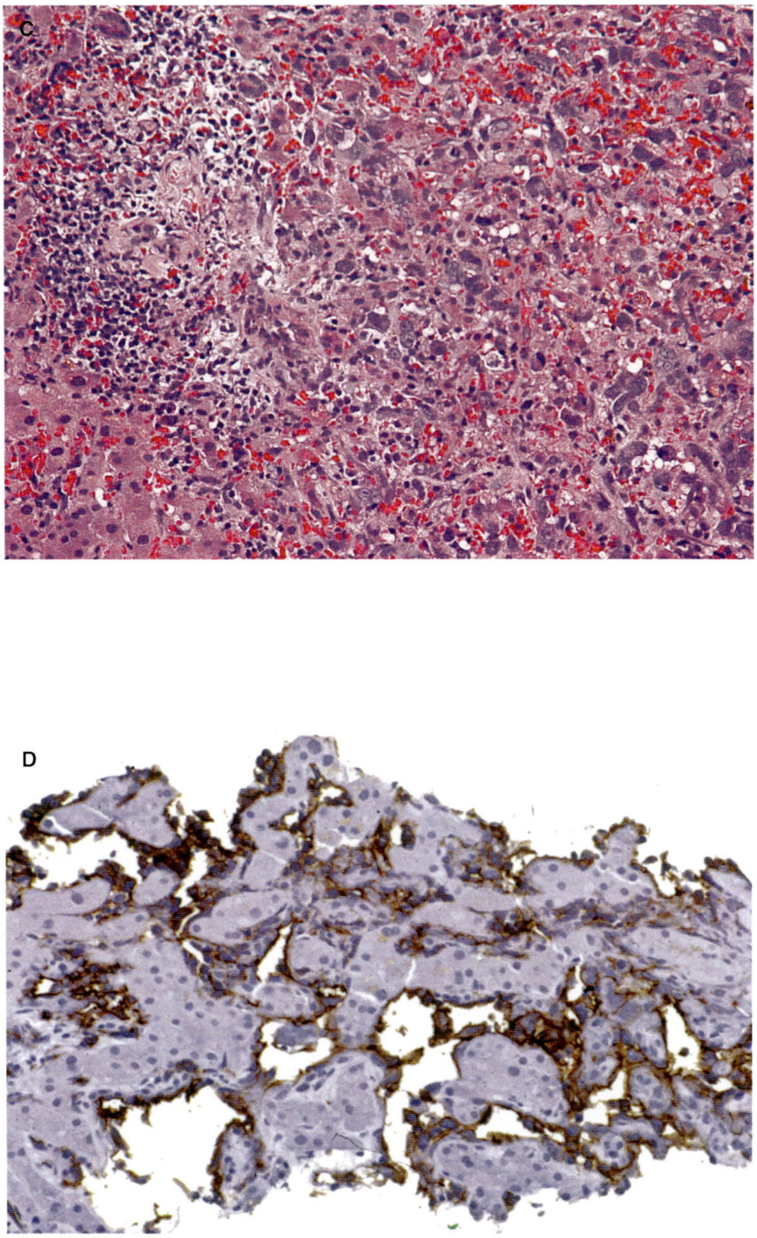

FIGURE 11-4

FIGURE 11-4 (C) Angiosarcoma with a more solid pattern. (D) Immunostain for factor VIII antigen.

12

Tumors With Mesenchymal Component

MESENCHYMAL HAMARTOMA

ANGIOMYOLIPOMA

HEPATOBLASTOMA

EMBRYONAL SARCOMA

Mesenchymal Hamartoma

DEFINITION

A benign liver lesion of childhood, with heterolgous mesenchymal elements; most cases discovered in the first 2 years of life, rare in children older than 5

CLINICAL FEATURES

- Male preponderance (2:1)
- Abdominal distention, palpable liver mass, or respiratory distress

PATHOLOGIC FEATURES

- Variable in size (rarely can reach up to 30 cm)
- Multiple cysts with clear, yellow, or gelatinous fluid (Figures 12-1A, B)
- Microscopically, primitive mesenchyme with entrapped bile ductules and hepatic parenchyma (Figures 12-1C, D)
- Spindle cells in a loose collagenous or myxoid stroma constitute the mesenchymal area (Figures 12-1C, D)

DIFFERENTIAL DIAGNOSIS

- Lymphangioma
- Infantile hemangioendothelioma

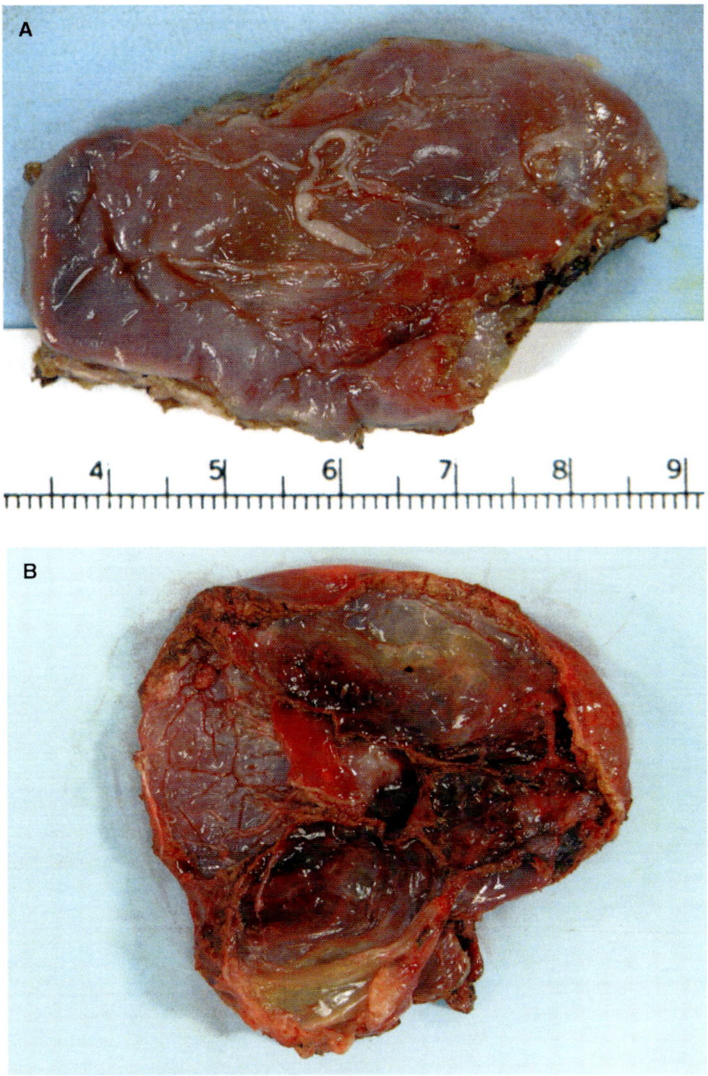

FIGURE 12-1

FIGURE 12-1 (A) Mesenchymal hamartoma. The resected tumor is well demarcated from adjacent parenchyma and has a cystic appearance. (B) Cut surface demonstrating multiple cysts with clear and gelatinous fluid, or dilated vascular areas and degenerative changes.

(*continued*)

Mesenchymal Hamartoma *(continued)*

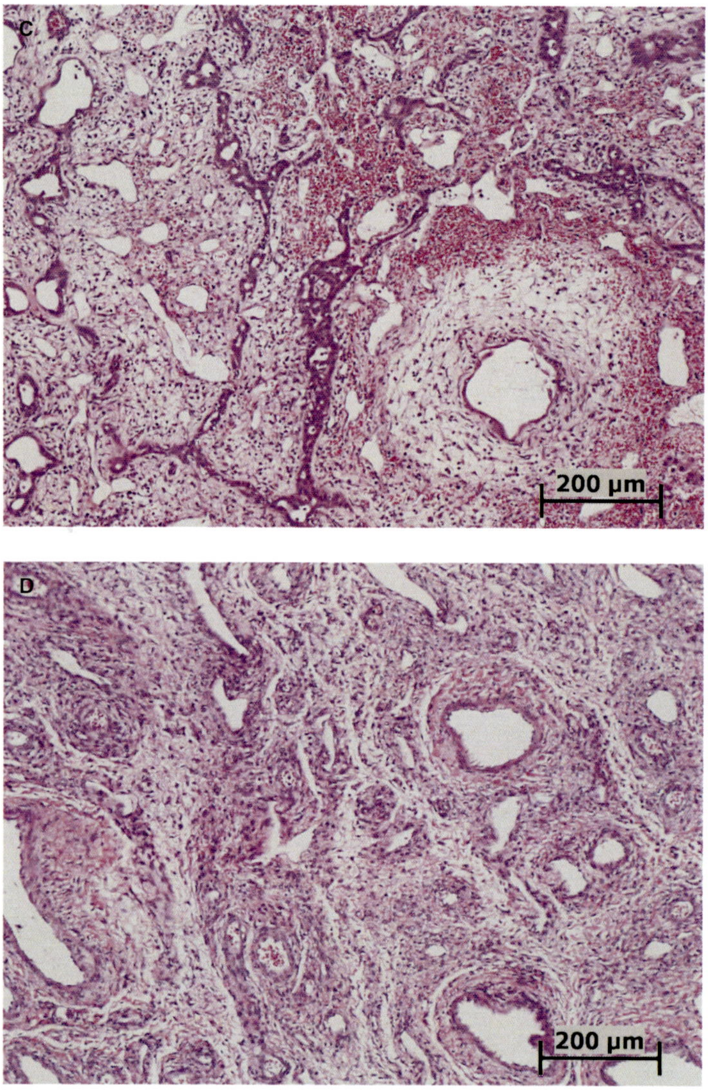

FIGURE 12-1

FIGURE 12-1 (C) Mesenchymal hamartoma. Loose connective tissue stroma with primitive sinusoid-like vascular spaces and ductules or cords of biliary epithelium.
(D) Mesenchymal hamartoma. Other areas contain mature venous and arterial blood vessels in a denser stroma, completely devoid of hepatocytes or biliary epithelia.

Angiomyolipoma

DEFINITION

A benign tumor (considered by some as a hamartomatous lesion), with a mixture of adipose and smooth muscle tissue and thick-walled blood vessels; thought to arise from perivascular epithelioid cells, thus considered part of the PEComa spectrum

CLINICAL FEATURES

- Young to middle-aged adults (fourth to fifth decade); more common in women
- Rarely associated with tuberous sclerosis
- Abdominal discomfort, fever, anorexia
- May present with rupture or hemorrhage due to large size

PATHOLOGIC FEATURES

- Usually solitary, large mass
- Cut surface yellow and soft to tan-white and firm
- Microscopic: mixture of mature adipose tissue, thick-walled blood vessels that are often hyalinized, and smooth muscle (Figures 12-2A, B)
- Smooth muscle component may be spindle or epithelioid; may grow in irregular prominent trabeculae
- Epithelioid cells characterized by round to polygonal shape and abundant eosinophilic cytoplasm; cytologic atypia may be seen (Figures 12-2A, B and C)
- Hematopoietic elements
- Some cases contain prominent lymphocytic infiltrate
- Immunostains positive for smooth muscle markers, HMB-45, and Melan-A; some positive for CD117 (Figure 12-2D)

DIFFERENTIAL DIAGNOSIS

- Hepatocellular adenoma or carcinoma (epithelioid smooth muscle cells)
- Gastrointestinal stromal tumor (CD117 positivity)
- Spindle cell sarcoma
- Metastatic melanoma

(continued)

Angiomyolipoma *(continued)*

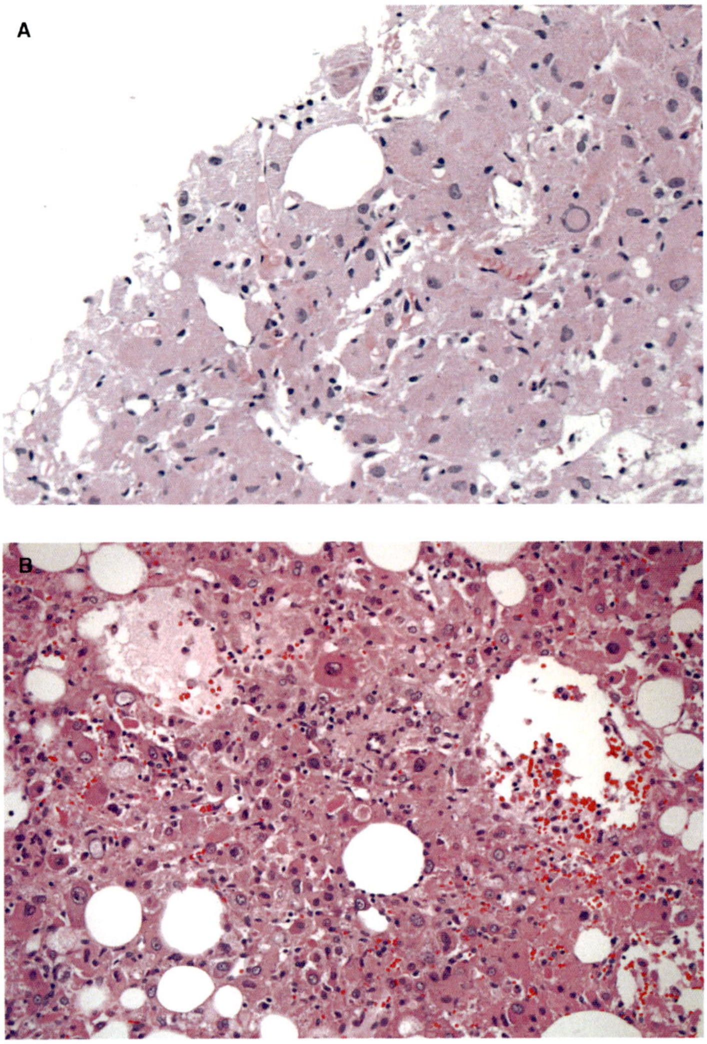

FIGURE 12-2

FIGURE 12-2 (A) Angiomyolipoma as seen in a core biopsy, consisting mainly of large epithelioid cells with abundant eosinophilic cytoplasm, small nuclei, and scant fat. (B) The resected specimen demonstrates more readily recognizable features of angiomyolipoma, with a mixture of epithelioid tumor cells and fat.

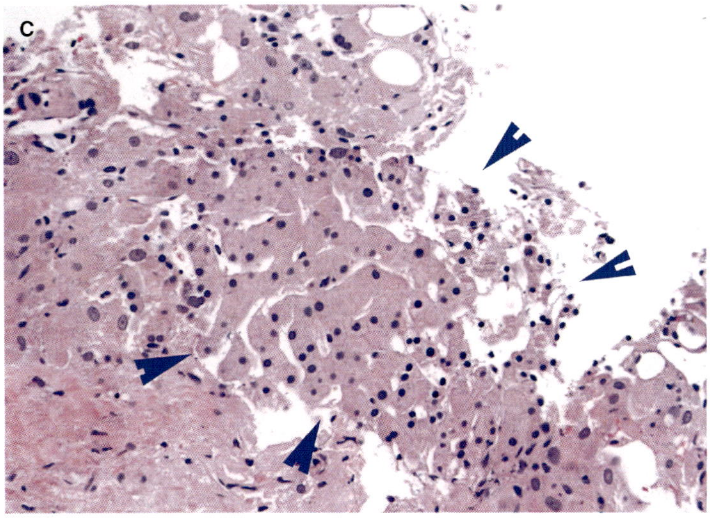

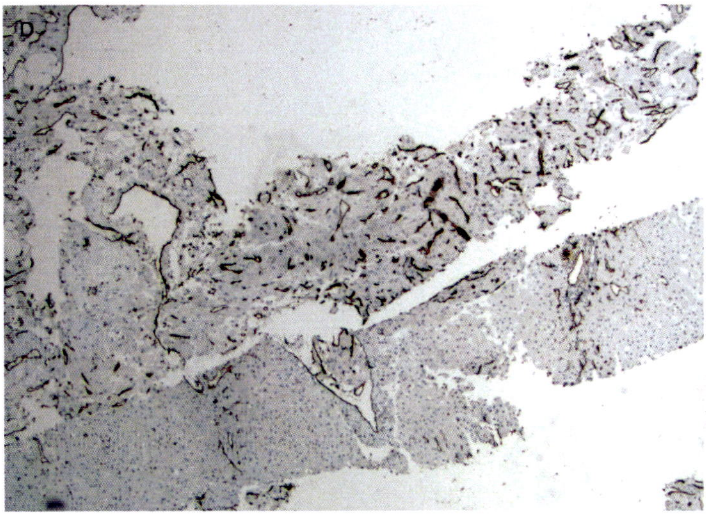

FIGURE 12-2

FIGURE 12-2 (C) Same case as Figure 12-2A. Other areas of the biopsy contain a cord of normal liver parenchyma (between arrowheads). Distinguishing between the tumor and normal hepatocytes relies on the better cord-like organization in the latter. (D) A CD34 immunostain highlights the endothelium of the sinusoidal network present in the background liver parenchyma, and the lack of sinusoids in the tumor.

Hepatoblastoma

DEFINITION

The most common pediatric malignant liver tumor, of blast cell origin; consisting of both epithelial and mesenchymal components

CLINICAL FEATURES

- Usually discovered in the first 3 years of life (90% diagnosed before age of 5); male-to-female ratio: 2 to 3:1
- May have other associated congenital anomalies: Beckwith-Wiedemann syndrome, glycogen storage disease, Down syndrome, familial polyposis coli, and rarely, precocious puberty (virilization)
- Presents with failure to thrive, abdominal mass, and weight loss
- Serum alpha fetoprotein (AFP) elevated
- Complete resection is treatment of choice (can be achieved in 40%–70% of cases)

PATHOLOGIC FEATURES

- A large single mass (up to 25 cm in largest dimension), multinodular with variegated cut surface and foci of hemorrhage or necrosis
- Some tumors contain only an epithelial component, with embryonal and fetal patterns in various combination; a small cell undifferentiated type also observed (Figure 12-3A)
- The mixed type contains epithelial and spindle cell mesenchymal elements, with osteoid-like material and other heterologous mesenchymal material, such as cartilage, striated muscle, or squamous epithelium (Figure 12-3B)
- *Embryonal pattern* less mature, with cords, trabeculae, ribbons, or acinar formation, small tumor cells with round nuclei and scant basophilic cytoplasm (Figures 12-3B, C)
- *Fetal pattern* characterized by tumor cells forming sheets, plates or thin cords, with a "light and dark" low power mosaic appearance due to alternating cells with fine granular cytoplasm or clear cytoplasm; most often associated with extramedullary hematopoiesis (Figure 12-3D)
- Mitoses rare in epithelial component
- Immunohistochemistry (IHC): reactive for HepPar-1, polyclonal CEA, alpha-fetoprotein, glypican-3, and chromogranin with variable degrees of expression
- May metastasize to lymph nodes, lung

DIFFERENTIAL DIAGNOSIS

- Hepatic adenoma (versus pure fetal hepatoblastoma)
- Hepatocellular carcinoma (versus pure fetal or macrotrabecular hepatoblastoma)
- Sarcoma (versus mixed epithelial-mesenchymal hepatoblastoma with teratoid features)
- Neuroblastoma (versus small cell undifferentiated hepatoblastoma)
- Hepatic adenoma
- Hepatocellular carcinoma

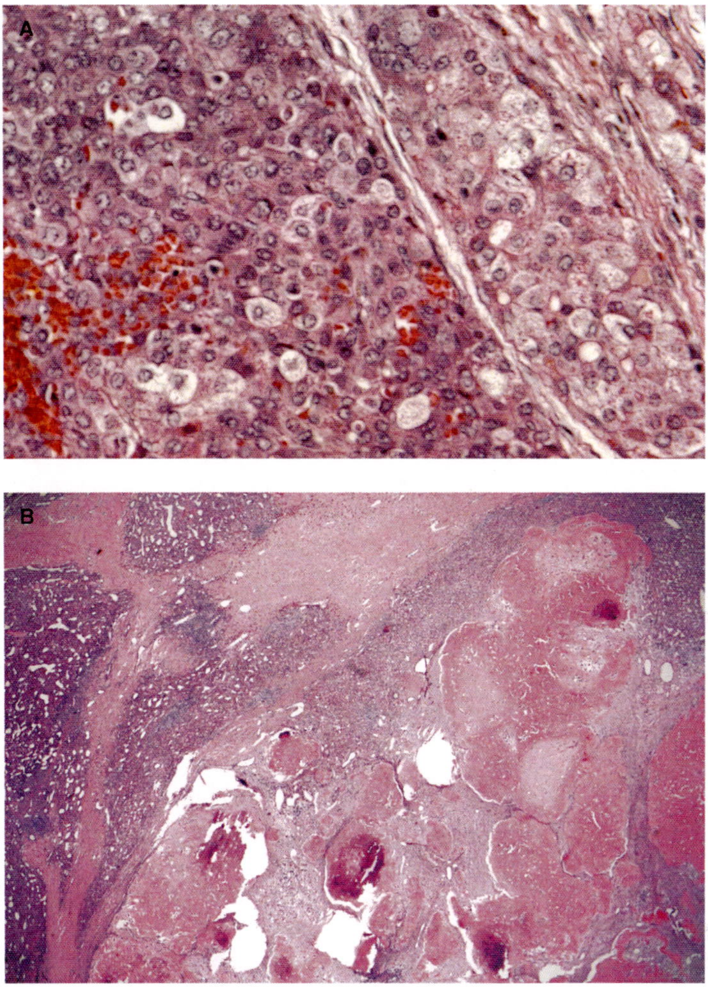

FIGURE 12-3

FIGURE 12-3 (A) Epithelial component in a mixed hepatoblastoma. Tumor cells resemble normal hepatocytes but with increased N/C ratio, and with a sheet-like arrangement. (B) Mixed epithelial mesenchymal type hepatoblastoma. Fibromyxoid and osteoid mesenchymal elements are evident. Nests of primitive epithelial component distributed in dense fibrous tissue.

(*continued*)

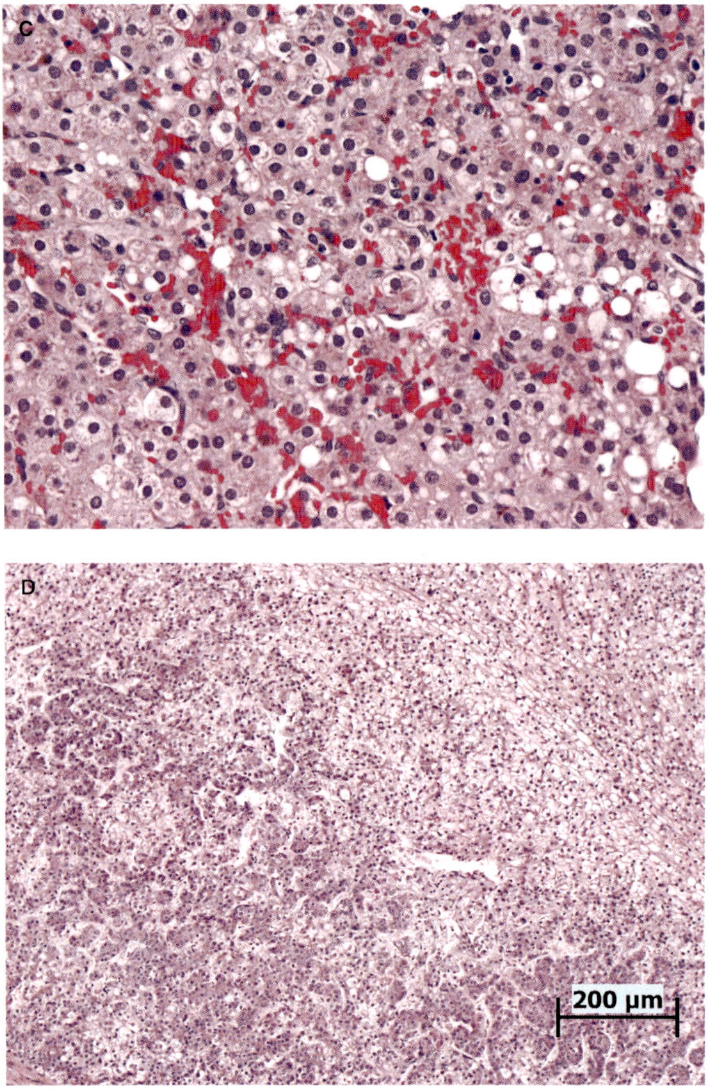

FIGURE 12-3

FIGURE 12-3 (C) Occasionally the epithelial component exhibits partial maturity, cytologically resembling differentiated hepatocytes but structurally remaining immature, mostly in sheets without cords. (D) Epithelial hepatoblastoma. The fetal type (right upper aspect) is characterized by sheets of cells with clear cytoplasm (glycogen-rich). The embryonal type (left lower aspect) is characterized by cords and rosettes of hepatocytes with more eosinophilic granular cytoplasm.

Embryonal Sarcoma

DEFINITION

Unique to the liver; rare and rapidly growing. Other names include undifferentiated sarcoma, mesenchymal sarcoma.

CLINICAL FEATURES

- Children and teenagers; mostly 6 to 10 years of age
- Abdominal swelling with or without palpable mass
- Abdominal pain
- Radiologically, large mass with solid and cystic components
- Treatment: combination of surgery and chemotherapy

PATHOLOGIC FEATURES

- Large mass (10–20 cm), with cystic degeneration and necrosis
- Cut surface: variegated, glistening, gray–white tissue, cystic areas with hemorrhage and/or necrosis
- Fibrous pseudocapsule
- Microscopic: large areas of necrosis; compactly or loosely arranged tumor cells in fibrous or abundant myxoid stroma (Figure 12-4A)
- Tumor cells stellate or spindle-shaped with indistinct cell outlines; hyperchromatic nuclei, brisk mitoses; bizarre giant cells (Figure 12-4B)
- Eosinophilic cytoplasmic globules (positive for periodic acid Schiff with diastase stain (PASD))

DIFFERENTIAL DIAGNOSIS

- Mesenchymal hamartoma

(*continued*)

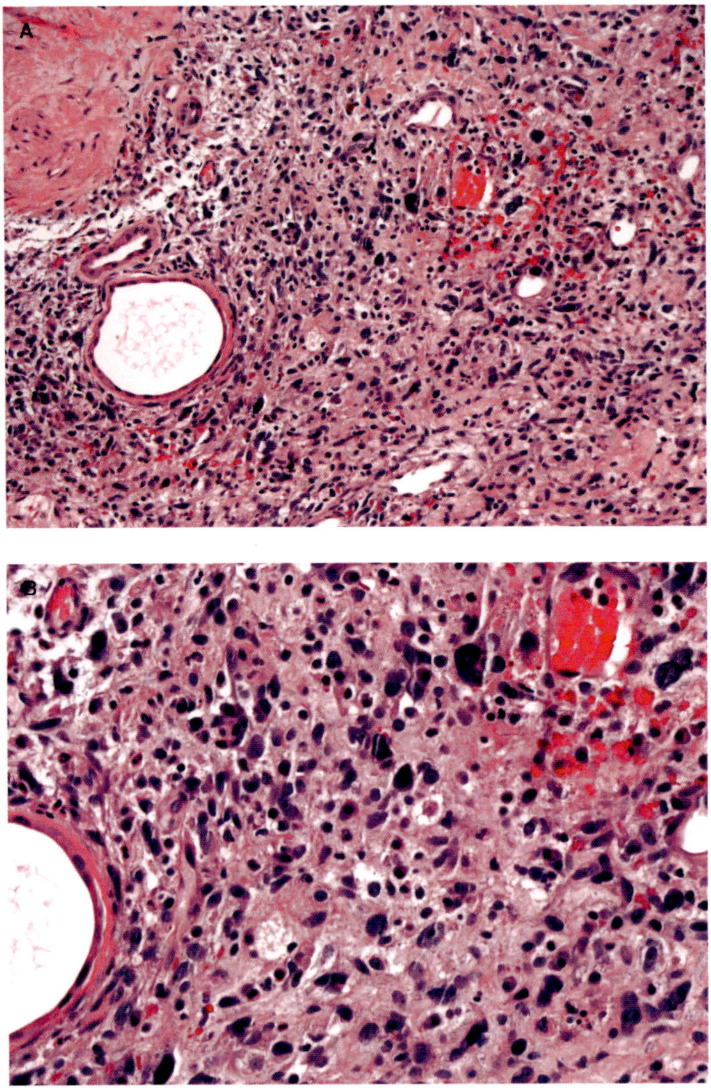

FIGURE 12-4

FIGURE 12-4 (A) Mesenchymal sarcoma. A large liver mass in a 14-year-old girl. Native parenchyma is replaced by spindle or epithelioid tumor cells, many with large hyperchromatic nuclei. Immunohistochemically these cells are negative for CAM5.2, AE1/AE3, myogenin, S-100, EGR, and CD31. (Picture courtesy of Dr. Xiuli Liu.) (B) Higher power view of Figure 12-4A). Cells with large bizarre nuclei are evident. (Picture courtesy of Dr. Xiuli Liu.)

Bibliography

CHAPTER 1. ACUTE HEPATITIS AND FULMINANT HEPATIC FAILURE

FULMINANT HEPATIC FAILURE

Bernal W, Auzinger G, Dhawan A, Wendon J. Acute liver failure. *Lancet.* 2010;376:190–201.

Lee WM, Squires RH Jr, Nyberg SL, Doo E, Hoofnagle JH. Acute liver failure: summary of a Workshop. *Hepatology.* 2008;47:1401–1415.

Stravitz RT, Lefkowitch JH, Fontana RJ, et al. Group Acute Liver Failure Study. Autoimmune acute liver failure: proposed clinical and histological criteria. *Hepatology.* 2011;53:517–526.

ACUTE HEPATOTROPIC VIRAL INFECTIONS

Johnson K, Kotiesh A, Boitnott JK, Torbenson M. Histology of symptomatic acute hepatitis C infection in immunocompetent adults. *Am J Surg Pathol.* 2007;31:1754–1758.

Liang TJ. Hepatitis B: the virus and disease. *Hepatology.* 2009;49:S13-S21.

Mushahwar IK. Hepatitis E virus: molecular virology, clinical features, diagnosis, transmission, epidemiology, and prevention. *J Med Virol.* 2008;80:646–658.

Okuno T, Sano A, Deguchi T, et al. Pathology of acute hepatitis A in humans. Comparison with acute hepatitis B. *Am J Clin Pathol.* 1984;81:162–169.

OTHER INFECTIOUS HEPATITIDES

Griffiths PD. Cytomegalovirus and the liver. *Semin Liver Dis.* 1984;4:307–313.

Sharma S, Mosunjac M. Herpes simplex hepatitis in adults: a search for muco-cutaneous clues. *J Clin Gastroenterol.* 2004;38:697–704.

Suh N, Liapis H, Misdraji J, Brunt EM, Wang HL. Epstein-Barr virus hepatitis: diagnostic value of in situ hybridization, polymerase chain reaction, and immunohistochemistry on liver biopsy from immunocompetent patients. *Am J Surg Pathol.* 2007;31:1403–1409.

FIBROSING CHOLESTATIC HEPATITIS

Davies SE, Portmann BC, O'Grady JG, et al. Hepatic histological findings after transplantation for chronic hepatitis B virus infection, including a unique pattern of fibrosing cholestatic hepatitis. *Hepatology.* 1991;13:150–157.

Dixon LR, Crawford JM. Early histologic changes in fibrosing cholestatic hepatitis C. *Liver Transpl.* 2007;13:219–226.

Satapathy SK, Sclair S, Fiel MI, Del Rio Martin J, Schiano T. Clinical characterization of patients developing histologically-proven fibrosing cholestatic hepatitis C post-liver transplantation. *Hepatol Res.* 2011;41:328–339.

Xiao SY, Lu L, Wang HL. Fibrosing cholestatic hepatitis: clinicopathologic spectrum, diagnosis and pathogenesis. *Int J Clin Exp Pathol.* 2008;1(5):396–402.

DRUG-INDUCED HEPATIC NECROSIS

Andrade RJ, Lucena MI, Kaplowitz N, et al. Outcome of acute idiosyncratic drug-induced liver injury: long-term follow-up in a hepatotoxicity registry. *Hepatology.* 2006;44:1581–1588.

Suzuki A, Brunt EM, Kleiner DE, et al. The use of liver biopsy evaluation in discrimination of idiopathic autoimmune hepatitis versus drug-induced liver injury. *Hepatology.* 2011;54:931–939.

PREGNANCY-RELATED ACUTE HEPATITIS

Hay JE. Liver disease in pregnancy. *Hepatology.* 2008;47:1067–1076.

Lee NM, Brady CW. Liver disease in pregnancy. *World J Gastroenterol.* 2009;15:897–906.

CHAPTER 2. CHRONIC HEPATITIS

CHRONIC VIRAL HEPATITIS

Brunt EM, Janney CG, Di Bisceglie AM, Neuschwander-Tetri BA, Bacon BR. Nonalcoholic steatohepatitis: a proposal for grading and staging the histological lesions. *Am J Gastroenterol.* 1999;94:2467–2474.

Intraobserver and interobserver variations in liver biopsy interpretation in patients with chronic hepatitis C. The French METAVIR Cooperative Study Group. *Hepatology.* 1994;20:15–20.

Ishak KG. Chronic hepatitis: morphology and nomenclature. *Mod Pathol.* 1994;7:690–713.

Knodell RG, Ishak KG, Black WC, et al. Formulation and application of a numerical scoring system for assessing histological activity in asymptomatic chronic active hepatitis. *Hepatology.* 1981;1:431–435.

Scheuer PJ. Classification of chronic viral hepatitis: a need for reassessment. *J Hepatol.* 1991;13:372–374.

GRANULOMATOUS HEPATITIS

Devaney K, Goodman ZD, Epstein MS, Zimmerman HJ, Ishak KG. Hepatic sarcoidosis. clinicopathologic features in 100 patients. *Am J Surg Pathol.* 1993;17:1272–1280.

Kleiner DE. Granulomas in the liver. *Semin Diagn Pathol.* 2006;23:161–169.

Lagana SM, Moreira RK, Lefkowitch JH. Hepatic granulomas: pathogenesis and differential diagnosis. *Clin Liver Dis.* 2010;14:605–617.

Snyder N, Martinez JG, Xiao S-Y. Chronic hepatitis C is commonly associated with hepatic granulomas. *World J Gastroenterol.* 2008;14(41):6366–6369.

Turhan N, Kurt M, Ozderin YO, Kurt OK. Hepatic granulomas: a clinicopathologic analysis of 86 cases. *Pathol Res Pract.* 2011;207:359–365.

AUTOIMMUNE HEPATITIS

Alvarez F, Berg PA, Bianchi FB, et al. International autoimmune hepatitis group report: review of criteria for diagnosis of autoimmune hepatitis. *J Hepatol.* 1999;31:929–938.

Czaja AJ, Bayraktar Y. Non-classical phenotypes of autoimmune hepatitis and advances in diagnosis and treatment. *World J Gastroenterol.* 2009;15:2314–2328.

Hennes EM, Zeniya M, Czaja AJ, et al, Group International Autoimmune Hepatitis. Simplified criteria for the diagnosis of autoimmune hepatitis. *Hepatology.* 2008;48:169–176.

Misdraji J, Thiim M, Graeme-Cook FM. Autoimmune hepatitis with centrilobular necrosis. *Am J Surg Pathol.* 2004;28:471–478.

Washington MK. Autoimmune liver disease: overlap and outliers. *Mod Pathol.* 2007;20 (suppl 1):S15–S30.

WILSON'S DISEASE

Gitlin JD. Wilson disease. *Gastroenterology.* 2003;125:1868–1877.

Stromeyer FW, Ishak KG. Histology of the liver in Wilson's disease: a study of 34 cases. *Am J Clin Pathol.* 1980;73:12–24.

DRUG-INDUCED HEPATITIS

Aithal PG, Day CP. The natural history of histologically proved drug induced liver disease. *Gut.* 1999;44:731–735.

Ramachandran R, Kakar S. Histological patterns in drug-induced liver disease. *J Clin Pathol.* 2009; 62:481–492.

PARASITIC INFESTATION

Gottstein B. Molecular and immunological diagnosis of echinococcosis. *Clin Microbiol Rev.* 1992;5:248–261.

Gryseels B, Polman K, Clerinx J, Kestens L. Human schistosomiasis. *Lancet.* 2006;368:1106–1118.

CHAPTER 3. BILIARY DISEASES AND CHOLESTASIS

BILIARY OBSTRUCTION AND ASCENDING CHOLANGITIS

Christoffersen P, Poulsen H. Histological changes in human liver biopsies following extrahepatic biliary obstruction. *Acta Pathol Microbiol Scand Suppl.* 1970;212(suppl 212):150+.

Lefkowitch JH. Histological assessment of cholestasis. *Clin Liver Dis.* 2004;8:27–40.

LIVER INVOLVEMENT IN SEPSIS

Banks JG, Foulis AK, Ledingham IM, Macsween RN. Liver function in septic shock. *J Clin Pathol.* 1982;35:1249–1252.

Lefkowitch JH. Bile ductular cholestasis: an ominous histopathologic sign related to sepsis and "cholangitis lenta." *Hum Pathol.* 1982;13:19–24.

PRIMARY BILIARY CIRRHOSIS (PBC)

Kaplan MM, Gershwin ME. Primary biliary cirrhosis. *N Engl J Med.* 2005;353:1261–1273.

Selmi C, Zuin M, Gershwin ME. The unfinished business of primary biliary cirrhosis. *J Hepatol.* 2008;49:451–460.

Washington MK. Autoimmune liver disease: overlap and outliers. *Mod Pathol.* 2007;20 (suppl 1):S15–S30.

PRIMARY SCLEROSING CHOLANGITIS

Bjornsson E, Chari ST, Smyrk TC, Lindor K. Immunoglobulin G4 associated cholangitis: description of an emerging clinical entity based on review of the literature. *Hepatology.* 2007;45:1547–1554.

Eaton JE, Talwalkar JA, Lazaridis KN, Gores GJ, Lindor KD. Pathogenesis of primary sclerosing cholangitis and advances in diagnosis and management. *Gastroenterology.* 2013;145:521–536.

Hirschfield GM, Karlsen TH, Lindor KD, Adams DH. Primary sclerosing cholangitis. *Lancet.* 2013;382:1587–1599.

Mendes F, Lindor KD. Primary sclerosing cholangitis: overview and update. *Nat Rev Gastroenterol Hepatol.* 2010;7:611–619.

OVERLAP SYNDROME

Beuers U. Hepatic overlap syndromes. *J Hepatol.* 2005;42 (suppl):S93–S99.

Chazouilleres O, Wendum D, Serfaty L, Montembault S, Rosmorduc O, Poupon R. Primary biliary cirrhosis-autoimmune hepatitis overlap syndrome: clinical features and response to therapy. *Hepatology.* 1998;28:296–301.

Suzuki Y, Arase Y, Ikeda K, et al. Clinical and pathological characteristics of the autoimmune hepatitis and primary biliary cirrhosis overlap syndrome. *J Gastroenterol Hepatol.* 2004;19:699–706.

Terracciano LM, Patzina RA, Lehmann FS, et al. A spectrum of histopathologic findings in autoimmune liver disease. *Am J Clin Pathol.* 2000;114:705–711.

CHAPTER 4. METABOLIC AND HEREDITARY DISORDERS

ALCOHOL-INDUCED LIVER DISEASE

Lefkowitch JH. Morphology of alcoholic liver disease. *Clin Liver Dis.* 2005;9:37–53.

Nakano M, Fukusato T. Histological study on comparison between NASH and ALD. *Hepatol Res.* 2005;33:110–115.

Sass DA, Shaikh OS. Alcoholic hepatitis. *Clin Liver Dis.* 2006;10:219–37, vii.

NONALCOHOLIC STEATOHEPATITIS

Brunt EM, Janney CG, Di Bisceglie AM, Neuschwander-Tetri BA, Bacon BR. Nonalcoholic steatohepatitis: a proposal for grading and staging the histological lesions. *Am J Gastroenterol.* 1999;94:2467–2474.

Kleiner DE, Brunt EM. Nonalcoholic fatty liver disease: pathologic patterns and biopsy evaluation in clinical research. *Semin Liver Dis.* 2012;32:3–13.

Kleiner DE, Brunt EM, Van Natta M, et al, Network Nonalcoholic Steatohepatitis Clinical Research. Design and validation of a histological scoring system for nonalcoholic fatty liver disease. *Hepatology.* 2005;41:1313–1321.

Ma H, Gomez V, Lu L, Yang X, Wu X, Xiao SY. Expression of adiponectin and its receptors in livers of morbidly obese patients with non-alcoholic fatty liver disease. *J Gastroenterol Hepatol.* 2009;24(2):233–237.

HEREDITARY HEMOCHROMATOSIS

Torbenson M. Iron in the liver: a review for surgical pathologists. *Adv Anat Pathol.* 2011;18:306–317.

ALPHA-1-ANTITRYPSIN DEFICIENCY

Fairbanks KD, Tavill AS. Liver disease in alpha 1-antitrypsin deficiency: a review. *Am J Gastroenterol.* 2008;103:2136–2141; quiz 42.

Stoller JK, Aboussouan LS. Alpha1-antitrypsin deficiency. *Lancet.* 2005;365:2225–2236.

CHAPTER 5. VASCULAR DISORDERS

NONCIRRHOTIC PORTAL HYPERTENSION

Chawla Y, Dhiman RK. Intrahepatic portal venopathy and related disorders of the liver. *Semin Liver Dis.* 2008;28:270–281.

Sarin SK, Kumar A, Chawla YK, et al, Members of the APASL Working Party on Portal Hypertension. Noncirrhotic portal fibrosis/idiopathic portal hypertension: APASL recommendations for diagnosis and treatment. *Hepatol Int.* 2007;1:398–413.

BUDD-CHIARI SYNDROME (HEPATIC VEIN THROMBOSIS)

Menon KV, Shah V, Kamath PS. The Budd-Chiari syndrome. *N Engl J Med.* 2004;350:578–585.

Valla DC. Primary Budd-Chiari syndrome. *J Hepatol.* 2009;50:195–203.

CARDIOGENIC HEPATIC CONGESTION

Giallourakis CC, Rosenberg PM, Friedman LS. The liver in heart failure. *Clin Liver Dis.* 2002;6: 947–967, viii-ix.

Naschitz JE, Slobodin G, Lewis RJ, Zuckerman E, Yeshurun D. Heart diseases affecting the liver and liver diseases affecting the heart. *Am Heart J*. 2000;140:111–120.

SINUSOIDAL OBSTRUCTION SYNDROME (VENO-OCCLUSIVE DISEASE)

DeLeve LD, Shulman HM, McDonald GB. Toxic injury to hepatic sinusoids: sinusoidal obstruction syndrome (veno-occlusive disease). *Semin Liver Dis*. 2002;22:27–42.

AMYLOIDOSIS

Buck FS, Koss MN. Hepatic amyloidosis: morphologic differences between systemic Al and Aa types. *Hum Pathol*. 1991;22:904–907.

Park MA, Mueller PS, Kyle RA, Larson DR, Plevak MF, Gertz MA. Primary (Al) hepatic amyloidosis: clinical features and natural history in 98 patients. *Medicine (Baltimore)*. 2003;82:291–298.

CHAPTER 6. NEONATAL DISORDERS

NEONATAL HEPATITIS

Balistreri WF. Neonatal cholestasis. *J Pediatr*. 1985;106(2):171–184.

Balistreri WF, Bezerra JA. Whatever happened to "neonatal hepatitis"? *Clin Liver Dis*. 2006;10(1):27–53, v.

Deorari AK, Broor S, Maitreyi RS, et al. Incidence, clinical spectrum, and outcome of intrauterine infections in neonates. *J Trop Pediatr*. 2000;46(3):155–159.

Kohnlein T, Welte T. Alpha-1 antitrypsin deficiency: pathogenesis, clinical presentation, diagnosis, and treatment. *Am J Med*. 2008;121(1):3–9.

Roberts EA. Neonatal hepatitis syndrome. *Semi Neonatol*. 2003;8(5):357–374.

PAUCITY OF INTRAHEPATIC BILE DUCTS

Alagille D, Estrada A, Hadchouel M, Gautier M, Odievre M, Dommergues JP. Syndromic paucity of interlobular bile ducts (Alagille syndrome or arteriohepatic dysplasia): review of 80 cases. *J Pediatr*. 1987;110(2):195–200.

Berezin S, Beneck D, Altman RP, Schwarz SM. Resolution of nonsyndromic paucity of intrahepatic bile ducts in infancy. *Dig Dis Sci*. 1995;40(1):82–85.

Hadchouel M. Paucity of interlobular bile ducts. *Semin Diagn Pathol*. 1992;9(1):24–30.

Hashida Y, Yunis EJ. Syndromatic paucity of interlobular bile ducts: hepatic histopathology of the early and endstage liver. *Pediatr Pathol*. 1988;8(1):1–15.

Hofmann JJ, Zovein AC, Koh H, Radtke F, Weinmaster G, Iruela-Arispe ML. Jagged1 in the portal vein mesenchyme regulates intrahepatic bile duct development: insights into Alagille syndrome. *Development*. 2010;137(23):4061–4072.

Kodama Y, Hijikata M, Kageyama R, Shimotohno K, Chiba T. The role of notch signaling in the development of intrahepatic bile ducts. *Gastroenterology*. 2004;127(6):1775–1786.

EXTRAHEPATIC BILIARY ATRESIA (EBA)

Morecki R, Glaser JH, Cho S, Balistreri WF, Horwitz MS. Biliary atresia and reovirus type 3 infection. *N Engl J Med*. 1982;307(8):481–484.

Rastogi A, Krishnani N, Yachha SK, Khanna V, Poddar U, Lal R. Histopathological features and accuracy for diagnosing biliary atresia by prelaparotomy liver biopsy in developing countries. *J Gastroenterol Hepatol*. 2009;24(1):97–102.

Vukovic J, Grizelj R, Bojanic K, et al. Ductal plate malformation in patients with biliary atresia. *Eur J Pediatr*. 2012;171(12):1799–1804.

CHAPTER 7. LIVER ALLOGRAFT PATHOLOGY

DONOR LIVER EVALUATION

Melin C, Miick R, Young NA, Ortiz J, Balasubramanian M. Approach to intraoperative consultation for donor liver biopsies. *Arch Pathol Lab Med.* 2013;137:270–274.

PRESERVATION INJURY

Zhai Y, Petrowsky H, Hong JC, Busuttil RW, Kupiec-Weglinski JW. Ischaemia-reperfusion injury in liver transplantation—from bench to bedside. *Nat Rev Gastroenterol Hepatol.* 2013;10:79–89.

ACUTE HUMORAL REJECTION

Hubscher SG. Antibody-mediated rejection in the liver allograft. *Curr Opin Organ Transplant.* 2012;17:280–286.

ACUTE CELLULAR REJECTION

Banff schema for grading liver allograft rejection: an international consensus document. *Hepatology.* 1997;25:658–663.

Demetris AJ, Ruppert K, Dvorchik I, et al. Real-time monitoring of acute liver-allograft rejection using the Banff schema. *Transplantation.* 2002;74:1290–1296.

Terminology for hepatic allograft rejection. International working party. *Hepatology.* 1995;22:648–654.

Tsamandas AC, Jain AB, Felekouras ES, Fung JJ, Demetris AJ, Lee RG. Central venulitis in the allograft liver: a clinicopathologic study. *Transplantation.* 1997;64:252–257.

CHRONIC REJECTION

Demetris A, Adams D, Bellamy C, et al. Update of the International Banff Schema for Liver Allograft Rejection: working recommendations for the histopathologic staging and reporting of chronic rejection. An International Panel. *Hepatology.* 2000;31:792–799.

Neil DA, Hubscher SG. Current views on rejection pathology in liver transplantation. *Transpl Int.* 2010;23:971–983.

GRAFT VERSUS HOST DISEASE (GVHD)

Cogbill CH, Drobyski WR, Komorowski RA. Gastrointestinal pathology of autologous graft-versus-host disease following hematopoietic stem cell transplantation: a clinicopathological study of 17 cases. *Mod Pathol.* 2011;24:117–125.

Quaglia A, Duarte R, Patch D, Ngianga-Bakwin K, Dhillon AP. Histopathology of graft versus host disease of the liver. *Histopathology.* 2007;50:727–738.

Shulman HM, Kleiner D, Lee SJ, et al. Histopathologic diagnosis of chronic graft-versus-host disease: National Institutes of Health Consensus Development Project on Criteria for Clinical Trials in Chronic Graft-Versus-Host Disease: II. Pathology Working Group Report. *Biol Blood Marrow Transplant.* 2006;12:31–47.

DE NOVO AUTOIMMUNE HEPATITIS

Fiel MI, Schiano TD. Plasma cell hepatitis (de-novo autoimmune hepatitis) developing post liver transplantation. *Curr Opin Organ Transplant.* 2012;17:287–292.

Guido M, Burra P. De novo autoimmune hepatitis after liver transplantation. *Semin Liver Dis.* 2011;31:71–81.

Heneghan MA, Portmann BC, Norris SM, et al. Graft dysfunction mimicking autoimmune hepatitis following liver transplantation in adults. *Hepatology.* 2001;34:464–470.

RECURRENT DISEASES

Hubscher SG. Recurrent and de-novo disease in the liver graft. *Curr Opin Organ Transplant.* 2006;11:283–288.

Petrovic LM. Recurrent disease following liver transplantation: current concepts. *Curr Opin Organ Transplant*. 2012;17:293–302.

Ruiz P, ed. *Transplantation Pathology*. 1st ed. Cambridge, UK: Cambridge University Press; 2009:152–166.

CHAPTER 8. LIVER INVOLVEMENT IN OTHER SYSTEMIC DISEASES

LYMPHOMA INVOLVING LIVER

Ferreri AJ, Govi S, Pileri SA. Hepatosplenic gamma-delta T-cell lymphoma. *Crit Rev Oncol Hematol*. 2012;83(2):283–292.

Lei KI. Primary non-Hodgkin's lymphoma of the liver. *Leuk Lymphoma*. 1998;29(3–4):293–299.

Noronha V, Shafi NQ, Obando JA, Kummar S. Primary non-Hodgkin's lymphoma of the liver. *Crit Rev Oncol Hematol*. 2005;53(3):199–207.

Salmon JS, Thompson MA, Arildsen RC, Greer JP. Non-Hodgkin's lymphoma involving the liver: clinical and therapeutic considerations. *Clin Lymphoma Myeloma*. 2006;6(4):273–280.

SYSTEMIC LUPUS ERYTHEMATOSUS

Efe C, Purnak T, Ozaslan E, et al. Autoimmune liver disease in patients with systemic lupus erythematosus: a retrospective analysis of 147 cases. *Scand J Gastroenterol*. 2011;46(6):732–737.

Fraenkel L, Simms RW. The clinical significance of liver disease in systemic lupus erythematosus. *J Clin Rheumatol*. 1996;2(1):23–28.

Irving KS, Sen D, Tahir H, Pilkington C, Isenberg DA. A comparison of autoimmune liver disease in juvenile and adult populations with systemic lupus erythematosus—a retrospective review of cases. *Rheumatology*. 2007;46(7):1171–1173.

Piga M, Vacca A, Porru G, Cauli A, Mathieu A. Liver involvement in systemic lupus erythematosus: incidence, clinical course and outcome of lupus hepatitis. *Clin Exp Rheumatol*. 2010;28(4):504–510.

CHAPTER 9. BENIGN EPITHELIAL NODULES AND TUMORS

FOCAL NODULAR HYPERPLASIA

Craig J, Peters R, Edmondson H. Benign tumors and tumor-like conditions. In: Hartmann W, Sobin L, eds. *Tumors of the Liver and Intrahepatic Bile Ducts*. Washington, DC: Armed Forces Institute of Pathology; 1989:8–98.

Ishak KG, Rabin L. Benign tumors of the liver. *Med Clin North Am*. 1975;59(4):995–1013.

Joseph NM, Ferrell LD, Jain D, et al. Diagnostic utility and limitations of glutamine synthetase and serum amyloid-associated protein immunohistochemistry in the distinction of focal nodular hyperplasia and inflammatory hepatocellular adenoma. *Mod Pathol*. 2014;27:62–72

Nguyen BN, Flejou JF, Terris B, Belghiti J, Degott C. Focal nodular hyperplasia of the liver: a comprehensive pathologic study of 305 lesions and recognition of new histologic forms. *Am J Surg Pathol*. 1999;23(12):1441–1454.

Wanless IR, Albrecht S, Bilbao J, et al. Multiple focal nodular hyperplasia of the liver associated with vascular malformations of various organs and neoplasia of the brain: a new syndrome. *Mod Pathol*. 1989;2(5):456–462.

Wanless IR, Mawdsley C, Adams R. On the pathogenesis of focal nodular hyperplasia of the liver. *Hepatology*. 1985;5(6):1194–1200.

HEPATIC ADENOMA

Bioulac-Sage P, Cubel G, Taouji S, et al. Immunohistochemical markers on needle biopsies are helpful for the diagnosis of focal nodular hyperplasia and hepatocellular adenoma subtypes. *Am J Surg Pathol*. 2012;36(11):1691–1699.

Bioulac-Sage P, Rebouissou S, Thomas C, et al. Hepatocellular adenoma subtype classification using molecular markers and immunohistochemistry. *Hepatology*. 2007;46(3):740–748.

Bluteau O, Jeannot E, Bioulac-Sage P, et al. Bi-allelic inactivation of TCF1 in hepatic adenomas. *Nat Genet*. 2002;32(2):312–315.
Cadoret A, Ovejero C, Terris B, et al. New targets of beta-catenin signaling in the liver are involved in the glutamine metabolism. *Oncogene*. 2002;21(54):8293–8301.
Craig J, Peters R, Edmondson H. Benign tumors and tumor-like conditions. In: Hartmann W, Sobin L, eds. *Tumors of the Liver and Intrahepatic Bile Ducts*. Washington, DC: Armed Forces Institute of Pathology; 1989:8–98.
De La Coste A, Romagnolo B, Billuart P, et al. Somatic mutations of the beta-catenin gene are frequent in mouse and human hepatocellular carcinomas. *Proc Natl Acad Sci USA*. 1998;95(15):8847–8851.
Ferrell LD. Hepatocellular carcinoma arising in a focus of multilobular adenoma. A case report. *Am J Surg Pathol*. 1993;17(5):525–529.
Torbenson M, Lee JH, Choti M, et al. Hepatic adenomas: analysis of sex steroid receptor status and the Wnt signaling pathway. *Mod Pathol*. 2002;15(3):189–196.
Zucman-Rossi J, Jeannot E, Nhieu JT, et al. Genotype-phenotype correlation in hepatocellular adenoma: new classification and relationship with HCC. *Hepatology*. 2006;43(3):515–524.

NODULAR REGENERATIVE HYPERPLASIA

Dill MT, Rothweiler S, Djonov V, et al. Disruption of Notch1 induces vascular remodeling, intussusceptive angiogenesis, and angiosarcomas in livers of mice. *Gastroenterology*. 2012;142(4):967–977, e2.
Fuss IJ, Friend J, Yang Z, et al. Nodular regenerative hyperplasia in common variable immunodeficiency. *Journal of Clinical Immunology*. 2013;33(4):748–758.
Reshamwala PA, Kleiner DE, Heller T. Nodular regenerative hyperplasia: not all nodules are created equal. *Hepatology*. 2006;44:7–14.
Rubbia-Brandt L, Lauwers GY, Wang H, et al. Sinusoidal obstruction syndrome and nodular regenerative hyperplasia are frequent oxaliplatin-associated liver lesions and partially prevented by bevacizumab in patients with hepatic colorectal metastasis. *Histopathology*. 2010;56(4):430–439.
Schouten JN, Garcia-Pagan JC, Valla DC, Janssen HL. Idiopathic noncirrhotic portal hypertension. *Hepatology*. 2011;54(3):1071–1081.
Ward C, Lucas M, Piris J, Collier J, Chapel H. Abnormal liver function in common variable immunodeficiency disorders due to nodular regenerative hyperplasia. *Clinical & Experimental Immunology*. 2008;153(3):331–337.

CHAPTER 10. MALIGNANT EPITHELIAL TUMORS

HEPATOCELLULAR CARCINOMA (HCC)

Craig J, Peters R, Edmondson H. Primary malignant epithelial tumors. In: Hartmann W, Sobin L, eds. *Tumors of the Liver and Intrahepatic Bile Ducts*. Washington, DC: Armed Forces Institute of Pathology; 1989:123–214.
Ferlay J, Shin HR, Bray F, Forman D, Mathers C, Parkin DM. Estimates of worldwide burden of cancer in 2008: GLOBOCAN 2008. *Int J Cancer*. 2010;127:2893–2917.
Koelma IA, Nap M, Huitema S, Krom RA, Houthoff HJ. Hepatocellular carcinoma, adenoma, and focal nodular hyperplasia. Comparative histopathologic study with immunohistochemical parameters. *Arch Pathol Lab Med*. 1986;110(11):1035–1040.
Lauwers GY, Terris B, Balis UJ, et al. Prognostic histologic indicators of curatively resected hepatocellular carcinomas: a multi-institutional analysis of 425 patients with definition of a histologic prognostic index. *Am J Surg Path*. 2002;26(1):25–34.
Yan BC, Gong C, Song J, et al. Arginase-1: a new immunohistochemical marker of hepatocytes and hepatocellular neoplasms. *Am J Surg Pathol*. 2010;34(8):1147–1154.

FIBROLAMELLAR HEPATOCELLULAR CARCINOMA (FLHC)

Abdul-Al HM, Wang G, Makhlouf HR, Goodman ZD. Fibrolamellar hepatocellular carcinoma: an immunohistochemical comparison with conventional hepatocellular carcinoma. *Int J Surg Pathol*. 2010;18(5):313-318.

Berman MA, Burnham JA, Sheahan DG. Fibrolamellar carcinoma of the liver: an immunohistochemical study of nineteen cases and a review of the literature. *Hum Pathol.* 1988;19(7):784–794.

Berman MM, Libbey NP, Foster JH. Hepatocellular carcinoma. Polygonal cell type with fibrous stroma–an atypical variant with a favorable prognosis. *Cancer.* 1980;46(6):1448–1455.

Craig JR, Peters RL, Edmondson HA, Omata M. Fibrolamellar carcinoma of the liver: a tumor of adolescents and young adults with distinctive clinico-pathologic features. *Cancer.* 1980;46(2):372–379.

Klein WM, Molmenti EP, Colombani PM, et al. Primary liver carcinoma arising in people younger than 30 years. *Am J Clin Pathol.* 2005;124(4):512–518.

Ross HM, Daniel HD, Vivekanandan P, et al. Fibrolamellar carcinomas are positive for CD68. *Mod Pathol.* 2011;24(3):390–395.

Wang JH, Dhillon AP, Sankey EA, Wightman AK, Lewin JF, Scheuer PJ. "Neuroendocrine" differentiation in primary neoplasms of the liver. *J Pathol.* 1991;163(1):61–67.

Ward SC, Huang J, Tickoo SK, Thung SN, Ladanyi M, Klimstra DS. Fibrolamellar carcinoma of the liver exhibits immunohistochemical evidence of both hepatocyte and bile duct differentiation. *Mod Pathol.* 2010;23(9):1180–1190.

INTRAHEPATIC CHOLANGIOCARCINOMA (ICC)

Aishima S, Kuroda Y, Nishihara Y, et al. Proposal of progression model for intrahepatic cholangiocarcinoma: clinicopathologic differences between hilar type and peripheral type. *Am J Surg Path.* 2007;31(7):1059–1067.

Chen MF. Peripheral cholangiocarcinoma (cholangiocellular carcinoma): clinical features, diagnosis and treatment [see comments]. *J Gastroenterol Hepatol.* 1999;14(12):1144–1149.

Chennat J, Konda VJ, Madrigal-Hoyos E, et al. Biliary confocal laser endomicroscopy real-time detection of cholangiocarcinoma. *Dig Dis Sci.* 2011;56(12):3701–3706.

Tihan T, Blumgart L, Klimstra DS. Clear cell papillary carcinoma of the liver: an unusual variant of peripheral cholangiocarcinoma [see comments]. *Hum Pathol.* 1998;29(2):196–200.

COMBINED HEPATOCELLULAR-CHOLANGIOCARCINOMA (CHCC)

Aishima S, Nishihara Y, Kuroda Y, et al. Histologic characteristics and prognostic significance in small hepatocellular carcinoma with biliary differentiation: subdivision and comparison with ordinary hepatocellular carcinoma. *Am J Surg Path.* 2007;31(5):783–791.

Maganty K, Levi D, Moon J, et al. Combined hepatocellular carcinoma and intrahepatic cholangiocarcinoma: outcome after liver transplantation. *Dig Dis Sci.* 2010;55(12):3597–3601.

Sasaki M, Nakanuma Y, Ho SB, Kim YS. Cholangiocarcinomas arising in cirrhosis and combined hepatocellular-cholangiocellular carcinomas share apomucin profiles. *Am J Clin Pathol.* 1998;109(3):302–308.

Tickoo SK, Zee SY, Obiekwe S, et al. Combined hepatocellular-cholangiocarcinoma: a histopathologic, immunohistochemical, and in situ hybridization study. *Am J Surg Path.* 2002;26(8):989–997.

Wakasa T, Wakasa K, Shutou T, et al. A histopathological study on combined hepatocellular and cholangiocarcinoma: cholangiocarcinoma component is originated from hepatocellular carcinoma. *Hepatogastroenterology.* 2007;54(74):508–513.

Yu XH, Xu LB, Zeng H, Zhang R, Wang J, Liu C. Clinicopathological analysis of 14 patients with combined hepatocellular carcinoma and cholangiocarcinoma. *Hepatobiliary Pancreat Dis Int.* 2011;10(6):620–625.

PRIMARY HEPATIC NEUROENDOCRINE TUMOR (PHNET)

Asakawa T, Tomioka T, Abe K, Yamaguchi T, Tsunoda T, Kanematsu T. Primary hepatic carcinoid tumor. *J Gastroenterol.* 1999;34(1):123–127.

Fenoglio LM, Severini S, Ferrigno D, et al. Primary hepatic carcinoid: a case report and literature review. *World J Gastroenterol.* 2009;15(19):2418–2422.

Iimuro Y, Deguchi Y, Ueda Y, et al. Primary hepatic carcinoid tumor with metachronous lymph node metastasis after long-term follow up. *J Gastroenterol Hepatol.* 2002;17(10):1119–1124.

Mehta DC, Warner RR, Parnes I, Weiss M. An 18-year follow-up of primary hepatic carcinoid with carcinoid syndrome. *J Clin Gastroenterol*. 1996;23(1):60–62.
Takayasu K, Muramatsu Y, Sakamoto M, et al. Findings in primary hepatic carcinoid tumor: US, CT, MRI, and angiography. *J Comput Assist Tomogr*. 1992;16(1):99–102.

METASTATIC CARCINOMA

Leong AS, Sormunen RT, Tsui WM, Liew CT. Hep Par 1 and selected antibodies in the immunohistological distinction of hepatocellular carcinoma from cholangiocarcinoma, combined tumours and metastatic carcinoma. *Histopathology*. 1998;33(4):318–324.
Terracciano LM, Glatz K, Mhawech P, et al. Hepatoid adenocarcinoma with liver metastasis mimicking hepatocellular carcinoma: an immunohistochemical and molecular study of eight cases. *Am J Surg Path*. 2003;27(10):1302–1312.
Ushiku T, Shinozaki A, Shibahara J, et al. SALL4 represents fetal gut differentiation of gastric cancer, and is diagnostically useful in distinguishing hepatoid gastric carcinoma from hepatocellular carcinoma. *Am J Surg Pathol*. 2010;34(4):533–540.
Xiao SY, Wang HL, Hart J, Fleming D, Beard MR. cDNA arrays and immunohistochemistry identification of CD10/CALLA expression in hepatocellular carcinoma. *Am J Pathol*. 2001;159(4):1415–1421.

CHAPTER 11. VASCULAR TUMORS

HEMANGIOMA

Ochsner JL, Halpert B. Cavernous hemangioma of the liver. *Surgery*. 1958;43(4):577–582.
Popescu I, Ciurea S, Brasoveanu V, et al. Liver hemangioma revisited: current surgical indications, technical aspects, results. *Hepatogastroenterology*. 2001;48(39):770–776.
Takagi H. Diagnosis and management of cavernous hemangioma of the liver. *Semin Surg Oncol*. 1985;1(1):12–22.

EPITHELIOID HEMANGIOENDOTHELIOMA

Burt A, Portmann B, Ferrell L. *MacSween's Pathology of the Liver*. 5th ed. Edinburgh, UK: Churchill Livingstone Elsevier; 2007.
Gray MH, Rosenberg AE, Dickersin GR, Bhan AK. Cytokeratin expression in epithelioid vascular neoplasms. *Hum Pathol*. 1990;21:212–217.

INFANTILE HEMANGIOENDOTHELIOMA

Cerar A, Dolenc-Strazar ZD, Bartenjev D. Infantile hemangioendothelioma of the liver in a neonate. Immunohistochemical observations. *Am J Surg Pathol*. 1996;20(7):871–876.
Marton T, Silhavy M, Csapo Z, Szende B, Papp Z. Multifocal hemangioendothelioma of the fetus and placenta. *Hum Pathol*. 1997;28(7):866–869.
Mo JQ, Dimashkieh HH, Bove KE. GLUT1 endothelial reactivity distinguishes hepatic infantile hemangioma from congenital hepatic vascular malformation with associated capillary proliferation. *Hum Pathol*. 2004;35(2):200–209.

ANGIOSARCOMA

Orlando G, Adam R, Mirza D, et al. Hepatic hemangiosarcoma: an absolute contraindication to liver transplantation–the European Liver Transplant Registry experience. *Transplantation*. 2013;95(6):872–877.
Smith PM, Williams DM, Evans DM, Path FR. Hepatic angiosarcoma in a vinyl chloride worker. *Bull N Y Acad Med*. 1976;52(4):447–452.
Wiland HO, Pai RK, Purysko AS. Hepatic angiosarcoma mimicking sinusoidal obstruction syndrome/venoocclusive disease: a pathologic-radiologic correlation. *Ann Diagn Pathol*. 2012;16(4):275–279.

CHAPTER 12. TUMORS WITH MESENCHYMAL COMPONENT

MESENCHYMAL HAMARTOMA

Chung EM, Cube R, Lewis RB, Conran RM. From the archives of the AFIP: pediatric liver masses: radiologic-pathologic correlation part 1. Benign tumors. *Radiographics.* 2010;30(3):801–826.

Cook JR, Pfeifer JD, Dehner LP. Mesenchymal hamartoma of the liver in the adult: association with distinct clinical features and histological changes. *Hum Pathol.* 2002;33(9):893–898.

Stocker JT. Hepatic tumors in children. *Clin Liver Dis.* 2001;5(1):259–281.

ANGIOMYOLIPOMA

Goodman ZD, Ishak KG. Angiomyolipomas of the liver. *Am J Surg Path.* 1984;8(10):745–750.

Makhlouf HR, Remotti HE, Ishak KG. Expression of KIT (CD117) in angiomyolipoma. *Am J Surg Path.* 2002;26(4):493–497.

Nonomura A, Enomoto Y, Takeda M, Takano M, Morita K, Kasai T. Angiomyolipoma of the liver: a reappraisal of morphological features and delineation of new characteristic histological features from the clinicopathological findings of 55 tumours in 47 patients. *Histopathology.* 2012;61(5):863–880.

Tsui WM, Colombari R, Portmann BC, et al. Hepatic angiomyolipoma: a clinicopathologic study of 30 cases and delineation of unusual morphologic variants. *Am J Surg Path.* 1999;23(1):34–48.

Tsui WM, Yuen AK, Ma KF, Tse CC. Hepatic angiomyolipomas with a deceptive trabecular pattern and HMB-45 reactivity. *Histopathology.* 1992;21(6):569–573.

HEPATOBLASTOMA

Abenoza P, Manivel JC, Wick MR, Hagen K, Dehner LP. Hepatoblastoma: an immunohistochemical and ultrastructural study. *Hum Pathol.* 1987;18(10):1025–1035.

Conran RM, Hitchcock CL, Waclawiw MA, Stocker JT, Ishak KG. Hepatoblastoma: the prognostic significance of histologic type. *Pediatr Pathol.* 1992;12(2):167–183.

Fasano M, Theise ND, Nalesnik M, et al. Immunohistochemical evaluation of hepatoblastomas with use of the hepatocyte-specific marker, hepatocyte paraffin 1, and the polyclonal anti-carcinoembryonic antigen. *Mod Pathol.* 1998;11(10):934–938.

Haas JE, Muczynski KA, Krailo M, et al. Histopathology and prognosis in childhood hepatoblastoma and hepatocarcinoma. *Cancer.* 1989;64(5):1082–1095.

Ruck P, Harms D, Kaiserling A. Neuroendocrine differentiation in hepatoblastoma. An immunohistochemical investigation. *Am J Surg Pathol.* 1990;14(9):847–855.

EMBRYONAL SARCOMA

Levy M, Trivedi A, Zhang J, et al. Expression of glypican-3 in undifferentiated embryonal sarcoma and mesenchymal hamartoma of the liver. *Hum Pathol.* 2012;43(5):695–701.

May LT, Wang M, Albano E, Garrington T, Dishop M, Macy ME. Undifferentiated sarcoma of the liver: a single institution experience using a uniform treatment approach. *J Pediatr Hematol Oncol.* 2012;34(3):e114-e116.

Shehata BM, Gupta NA, Katzenstein HM, et al. Undifferentiated embryonal sarcoma of the liver is associated with mesenchymal hamartoma and multiple chromosomal abnormalities: a review of eleven cases. *Pediatr Dev Pathol.* 2011;14(2):111–116.

Index